HUGE IN HIGH SCHOOL™

FITNESS FOR *LIFE*

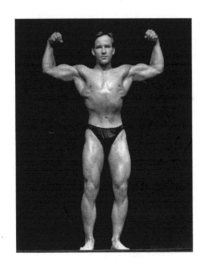

G.C. Schop

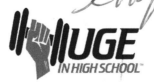

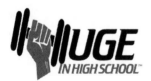

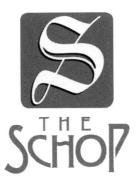

THE
SCHOP

The online website gains you access to books for sale as well as various blogs written to and for readers. Keep in touch, ask questions, download free content, and discover more about the author.

VISIT **THESCHOP.COM**

*FOR JACKSON AND CONOR,
AND FOR ALL BOYS GROWING UP
TO BE MEN.*

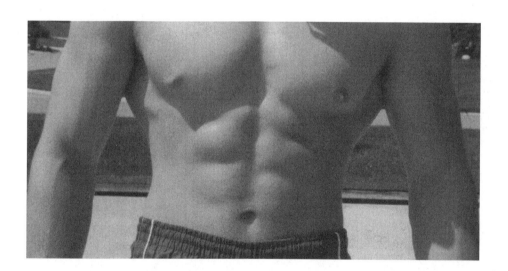

CONTENTS

1. INTRODUCTION 9

"Read this entire book before you do anything."

2. MIND 15

"Slow down. Reread this book before you start exercising."

3. DIET + MIND 29

"The fuel you choose to run your body."

12. APPENDICES 121

"Fill in the Blanks to Solve the Riddle."

1.

INTRODUCTION

"Read this entire book before you do anything."

ACKNOWLEDGEMENTS

I want to thank all the great people I met in the gym as a teenager and, of course, V.P. who first introduced me to weight training in the original dungeon in West Bloomfield, Michigan. I'd also like to thank my favorite bodybuilders of the '70s who inspired me and continue to motivate me throughout my life.

While no one is perfect, young people need role models that appear, at times, unimaginable, nonetheless very real; we thank these foundations, these mothers and fathers of our time, now, before, and afterward.

WELCOME

If you are a freshman in high school, you've been in school for about ten years, seven hours each day.

Have you spent ten years working on your body? Even one hour per day? Do you even walk much?

If you want to be strong, muscular, and fit for life, then it's time to start a **Huge in High School**™ workout program. And NO, you don't have to be in high school to benefit from this book, but the earlier you start the better.

The information to follow will save you years of trial-and-error and countless hours on the Internet looking for a miracle pill, formula, or workout program.

WHAT'S IN THIS BOOK?

This is a short book with just enough words, pictures, and all the BASIC information you need to understand and follow a **Huge in High School**™ workout program and a **Huge in High School**™ diet and schedule. This book is both simple and philosophical, and it is based on three decades of personal experience starting from age twelve. The most important ingredient in this book is YOU.

WHAT'S NOT IN THIS BOOK?

Information on any muscle enhancement drugs (legal or illegal) is not included in this book. At this point in my life (2016), I have never taken any enhancement drugs such as steroids, or any similar substance for that matter; therefore, I have no real knowledge to share in this area.

Steroids and other enhancement drugs are often a requirement for professional bodybuilders. Having only competed as a teenager, I was clueless about the real world of competitive bodybuilding and really never had the intention of taking anything.

In the future, it is possible that certain drugs may develop into possible fountains of youth for the human body. As of now, however, I think a solid argument can be made for staying away from all these types of drugs, especially during the youthful and healthiest years of the human life span.

TRAINING PHILOSOPHY

A young person needs practice exploring his or her physical powers while learning to open up the mind to think.

As babies, we thrive on physical contact, and as we progress throughout the stages toward adulthood, we work our mind and body, for the most part unfocused and easily distracted. Even as young adults, "stuff" such as school and part-time employment can lead us astray from ourselves (this only gets worse as we become adults), leaving our bodies and minds to detach and weaken from lack of use and focus. We become machines that do rather than experience, grow, and transcend.

No one's path is the same, but in order to help attain clarity, stability, growth, and emotional balance, one must move muscle.

I am one man, one life, on one adventure. Every single human being is unique. Each of us must find our own path and balance both mentally and physically. I offer thirty years of experience and what I believe people of almost any age need: knowledgeable guidance toward a healthy physical training program. Thank you for taking this journey with me in revealing the mystery of lifting weights, bringing us all closer to solving the riddle of iron.

WARNINGS

SEE YOUR PHYSICIAN BEFORE beginning any exercise program and/or changing your physical activity patterns.

Always consult with your doctor or physician, particularly if you are inactive, overweight, and/or suffer from any sort of medical condition that could potentially worsen with exercise.

It is always important to start a serious exercise program SLOWLY.

This book includes advice on exercise and diet from real-life experience, and is an exact organized blueprint of what I did to gain muscle and strength as well as to continue onward in a happy and healthy lifestyle.

RISKS

Since I was interested in competition bodybuilding at a young age, I chose to push my body to its limits while trying to do it as safely as possible. A young body is very forgiving, but this isn't the case when you get older. In weightlifting, the RISK increases as you increase the amount of time you exercise each body part and the amount of weight you use.

The information to follow will help you choose what type of **Huge in High School**™ workout program is right for you. I suggest any long-term, lifelong program because it attains what I call The *Real* Goal. I feel obligated, however, to provide information on what I believe is the maximum amount of training one can do at a young age versus an older age range. This way you will learn more about YOUR body and decide what level of intensity is best for it and for YOU.

WORKING OUT ALONE

Although it might seem glorious to "die on the bench" like some sort of chivalrous knight or modern day warrior, it is much safer to have someone else around. There are safe ways to weight train *without* a partner; however, it is probably smarter to exercise around other people, such as gym members or, at the very least, make sure someone else is in the house while you work out. You never know if and when you'll need assistance.

I'm sure you've heard of people that drop barbells on themselves and cannot get them off; this is why dumbbells are best when lifting alone.

If you're not a listener, here are a few tips and suggestions (not guarantees) to stay alive whenever using barbells alone:

1)   Do NOT use clips or locks on the end of each side of the bar. These clips will stop the weight from sliding off the bar onto the floor. If you are ever stuck or pinned under the barbell, you can simply tip the bar to the left or right (whichever you prefer during this state of panic) allowing all the weight to drop to the floor, but be READY for the bar to tip quickly the other way as the other side's weight will undoubtedly want to come off! I've seen it happen in the gym. It looks like the person is kayaking on his or her back using an Olympic-sized straight bar as the paddle.

2)   In the event that you left the clips or lock ON, the best chance you have (besides screaming for help) is to dump the bar to the left or right and then slowly inch your way off the bench while trying to hold the bar from crushing your chest and rib cage.

3)   Do NOT try to roll the barbell down over your stomach and genital area. While this will probably work with lighter weight, I can only imagine that heavier weight will be the death of you.

This book will navigate you through all the amateur pitfalls that are humanly possible. Great effort has been made to pay attention to every minor detail. While no one can teach *everything* there is regarding individual exercise and weight training, I will do my best to answer this ancient riddle of iron.

GENDER

Both males and females can benefit from weight training and exercise. As a male, however, my scope has its limits due to my gender and experience.

AGE

It is up to you to consult a physician, evaluate your body, and make an educated decision on when and how to start exercising. I started around age twelve. Good or bad, there's a lot of information regarding when and how to start exercising. Like most stuff, I imagine it depends on a number of factors. If you're in absolute fear of causing damage to your body while you're growing, you may want to stick with body weight exercises until you're fully grown. Again, I recommend doing some research on what's right for you. In the end, it's your decision.

AGE OVER FORTY

If you're reading this book and you're forty or over, it's not a problem at all. Just make sure you pay attention to which workouts you're choosing to do. There will be occasional references to certain exercises that have been suggested by some surgeons to avoid after age forty. The suggestions may surprise you, but as always, you can decide for yourself. Another obvious adjustment to your workout program is making sure you have enough time for the body to heal between workouts and to consider how much heavy lifting you do. An older joint and muscle structure can have its limits and weak points, but that doesn't mean you can't look and feel great, even if you're a beginner at an older age.

PUSH-UPS AND PULL-UPS BEYOND AGE FORTY?

Here are the two exercises that made the list that will surprise you. Despite Internet videos of eighty- and ninety-year-old men doing push-ups and pull-ups, it has still been suggested by some shoulder surgeons NOT to do these two classic exercises past age forty or so.

The suggestion is that one should avoid the pull-up because tendons lose elasticity as we age past forty. This increases the chance of tearing a tendon because this exercise requires so much more stabilization of the joint area vs. the "Lat Pull-down" machine where you're obviously not balancing and holding up your body weight.

Likewise, the push-up could be replaced indefinitely by the dumbbell press for the same reasons stated above regarding pull-ups.

Either way, it will be up to you when the time comes . . .

MIND

"Slow down. Reread this book before you start exercising."

THE *REAL* GOAL

Using your muscles leads to discipline and focus in your life. Your daily workout trains your mind to focus, think, plan, and dream.

This should be your only goal because it is important to think about your WHOLE life. You want to be able to exercise your ENTIRE life, not just when you're young. It doesn't make sense to go to extremes and destroy your body. YOU control the exercises; the exercises don't control you.

EVERYTHING else is a SIDE-EFFECT that will probably INCREASE the following:

- muscles
- strength
- health and wellness
- charisma
- self-confidence
- attention from love interests
- quality of life
- social life
- energy
- wealth and opportunity
- emotional and physical balance
- overall happiness
  . . . and the list goes on . . .

Exercise helps your life "workout."

WHO AM I? DOES IT MATTER?

It seems anytime you buy something nowadays, especially in regards to fitness, the spokesperson better be the best of the best: extremely low body-fat, overly charismatic, a model, an almost picture-perfect example of fitness.

While being a positive role model helps, there are other factors besides being in great shape. While it can be tempting to choose a role model or personal trainer based on looks and external factors, it should be noted that if your objective is to LEARN from that person, personality, intelligence, and one's ability to teach you are also important.

I'm the guy on the cover of this book (1991) from when I was in high school, some twenty-five years ago from its publication. Six feet two inches tall? 220 pounds? No way! At the time of this book cover's picture (age seventeen), my contest weight was about 155 pounds at five feet six and a half inches!

HIGH SCHOOL TEENAGE BODYBUILDER MEASUREMENTS

AGE	18	BICEPS	17 inches
HEIGHT	5' 6–1/2" inches	WAIST	32 inches
WEIGHT	171 pounds	LEGS	23 inches
CHEST	44 inches	CALVES	17 inches

- 3rd place Teenage Michigan Bodybuilding Contest (1991)
- 300-pound bench press (1 time)*
- 315-pound squat (4 times deep to the ground)*
- * low-rep maximum exertions of strength and extended range of motion can be dangerous and unnecessary

AFTER HIGH SCHOOL

- American Council on Exercise (ACE) Certified Fitness Trainer (Age 20)
- Lifting and staying in shape to the best of my ability ever since

A RELIC PAGE FROM THE ANCIENT
TRAINING DIARY "BENCH PRESS"

Although I absolutely do NOT recommend one-rep maximums, I lacked the knowledge of its possible negative side-effects. Therefore, here is my REAL example of how you can INCREASE in STRENGTH over time. Again, you could just as easily write down weight you successfully lift for four reps vs. one rep in order to track your performance.

DATE	AGE	BENCH PRESS	BAR
July 8, 1988	14	160 lbs.	6 feet
July 27, 1988	14	165 lbs.	6 feet
August 15, 1988	14	175 lbs.	6 feet
September 18, 1988	14	180 lbs.	6 feet
October 30, 1988	14	185 lbs.	6 feet
February 9, 1989	15	190 lbs.	6 feet
August 5, 1989	15	200 lbs.	7 feet
August 13, 1989	15	205 lbs.	7 feet
August 27, 1989	15	210 lbs.	7 feet
September 10, 1989	15	215 lbs.	7 feet
September 17, 1989	15	220 lbs.	7 feet
October 1, 1989	15	225 lbs.	7 feet
July 26, 1990	16	235 lbs.	7 feet
September 19, 1990	16	240 lbs.	7 feet
October 6, 1990	16	245 lbs.	7 feet
February 1, 1991	17	250 lbs.	7 feet
April 18, 1991	17	260 lbs.	7 feet
July 28, 1991	17	270 lbs.	7 feet
March 27, 1992	18	300 lbs.	7 feet

CERTIFIED PERSONAL TRAINER

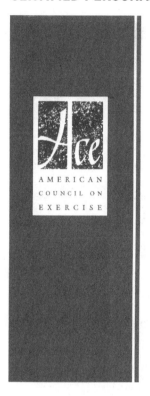

American Council on Exercise

CERTIFIED PERSONAL TRAINER

This is to certify that

Gregory C. Schop

*has successfully demonstrated written competency to design and
implement fitness programs to healthy persons who have no apparent
physical limitations or special medical needs.*

August 31, 1996
Valid Through

Executive Director

Okay, so what? Obviously I've spent a good portion of my life lifting weights and learning. In the end, I inherited some pretty good muscle from my parents (GENETICS). Not everyone will attain these feats of strength at a weight of 155 pounds, but I also guarantee there is someone out there that will! Stronger! Bigger! There will always be someone bigger and stronger. It isn't about THAT because once you hit age 100, there's no way you'll be the strongest anymore, even if you used to be.

DON'T BE A MEATHEAD

FORGET THE MEATHEAD STATS!!! (I know this because I was a meathead at one time.) You have to make sure you don't get TOO into your body. My face says it all. Here I am at 17.

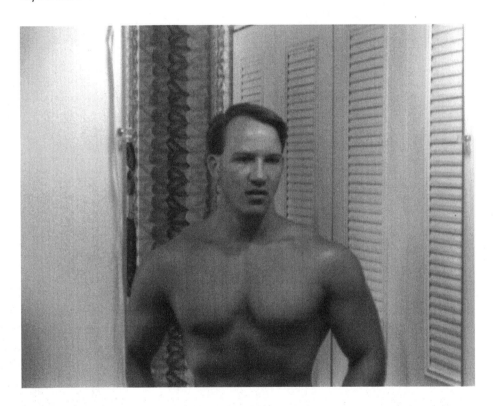

You have a MIND, you have a BODY, and around 2,500 years ago, the society of Ancient Greece recognized and honored this relationship: the mind and body go together.

DOES YOURS?

TOO MANY DETAILS

There are seemingly endless amounts of fitness information that you can look up on the Internet. If you spent half of that time working out, you'd be ahead of the game. There are endless details that might be nice to know, but they're unnecessary, and in many cases just get in the way, leading to overthinking and overtraining. If you want to be a doctor or you want to pass a fitness trainer test, then I'm afraid you'll have to learn ALL these words and many more:

Lactic acid—VO2 MAX—MaxOT—Isolation—Isometric—Plyometric

Latissimus Dorsi—Glutes—Endomorph—Mesomorph—Ectomorph—Ketosis

Pectoral—Traps—Pecs—Metabolism—Quads—Hams—Bis—Tris

Diastolic—Aerobic—Anaerobic—Cross-training—Resistance—Glycogen

Electrolytes—Systolic—Serrated—Ligament—Negatives—Amino acid

Glutamine—Creatine—Anabolic steroids—Basal metabolic rate (BMR)

Cardiorespiratory—Cardiovascular—Vascularity—Beats per minute (bpm)

Hydration—Dehydration

But . . . you will probably learn a few of them anyway . . .

FOUR MYTHS

1) "You can get huge *just like me.*"
(*Maybe* if it's your twin.)

2) "I got big by taking/using _____."
(Many supplements and pieces of gym equipment are a waste of money.)

3) "The secret to working out is . . . "
(What secret? There are only basic principles and rules.)

4) "My workout is the greatest . . ."
(What's good for you might not be good for someone else's mind and body.)

FOUR TRUTHS

#1 THE TRUTH YOU *DON'T* WANT TO HEAR

Your PARENTS (genetics) matter. The amount of muscle, the type of muscle, where all that stuff attaches to your bones, the length of your arms, your height, your eye color, hair color . . . everything comes from your parents and their parents . . . and it all leads to this:

Not everyone can attain the SAME size and strength, but ALL of us can INCREASE size and strength.

#2 THE TRUTH YOU *NEED* TO HEAR

There is NOT only one way to work out. Once you realize that, you start to understand that YOU are the one who needs to take charge of your own workouts and life. Everything being taught in this book comes from MY experience, so it is important to remember that you're going to benefit a ton from this book because you will be learning HOW to apply MY experience to YOUR body and life. Then and only then will it become YOUR experience.

#3 THE TRUTH ABOUT PILLS, POWDERS, AND MAGICAL POTIONS

Don't kid yourself. You need healthy FOOD and clean WATER. *From ages thirteen to forty, I NEVER took any supplements!* All the pictures you see in this book are supplement free. It wasn't until my forties that I tried taking an ALL NATURAL, low calorie WHEY PROTEIN powder, using it only after intense weightlifting workouts. While I feel whey protein is safe in limited quantities, some supplements can cause issues, and I STRONGLY caution that you READ about all the negative side-effects BEFORE you start taking them. It's difficult to measure if any gains or performance is from the supplement rather than the lifting itself. Currently, I am back to just food, water, and exercising.

#4 THE TRUTH ABOUT WHAT YOU NEED TO GET BIGGER AND/OR STRONGER

At the end of the day, all you really need is YOUR BODY. The only reason to use weights is to go beyond your body weight. When you go beyond your body weight, the muscles need to get stronger (maybe even bigger) to handle the extra weight load. It can be argued that you do NOT need to use weights. Keeping in shape using your body is perfectly acceptable, but let's face it, a lot of people want to challenge their body! If the body has the ability to grow bigger and stronger, then why not make it do so? It's all up to YOU. Bodyweight exercises and/or exercises using weights are BOTH an acceptable choice. Remember The *Real* Goal.

THE IMPORTANT STUFF YOU "NEED"

The only thing you really *need* when working out is your mind and BODY. You can run in place, drop to do a bunch of push-ups, jump up to do some pull-ups on whatever will hold your weight, leap up and down onto a table or bench from the floor, and once you're exhausted, lying on the ground, whip off a few abdominal crunches and then call it a workout. Done. Believe it or not, doing just *that* will get you into better shape. There are numerous activities that will keep your body moving: martial arts sparring, boxing, jumping rope, swimming, running, walking, loading boxes onto trucks, gymnastics, golfing (no cart, though), jumping jacks, and pretty much anything you can think up.

It all depends on your personal goal. Since you're reading this book, you probably want to get in shape and build muscle and strength. Sure, some of that stuff mentioned above can do that, but if your goal is building a bigger and stronger foundation of muscle for the future (beyond using just your body weight), then you'll need a few more things. Read on.

THINGS YOU NEED FOR MUSCLE AND STRENGTH BEYOND YOUR BODY WEIGHT (HOME)

When building muscle and strength beyond using your body weight, resistance or weights are required in some form or another.

If you're going to use weights, the cheapest way to do so (and perhaps the best way) is to buy the following items:

1) A FLAT WEIGHT BENCH

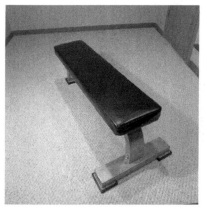

It should be solid and stable with a thick and firm cushion. Don't go cheap on this item. You always want a safe and stable surface as your "partner" and foundation. You don't have to buy a commercial gym bench, but the closer to that type of stability the better. The bench shown costs a little over $200, whereas commercial would probably be double or triple. This bench is very stable for the price.

2) DUMBBELLS

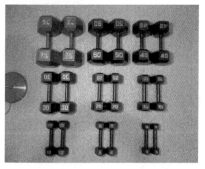

Basic, solid dumbbells of any type are best. Unfortunately, the stronger you get, the more money you'll have to spend on heavier dumbbells. You can get fancy with these and spend a TON of cash, but it isn't necessary. For example, buying dumbbells in increments of 10s, 20s, 30s, 40s, and 50s . . . will save you money.

3) PULL-UP BAR (PURCHASED OR HOMEMADE)

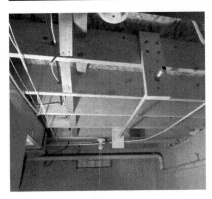

If you can't do ONE pull-up, then you'll either need someone to "spot" you by pushing you up by your legs or you'll need a "lat" pull-down machine or a similar machine that assists or copies the pull-up exercise. You could leave this exercise out of your workout, of course, but it has some major advantages in strengthening your body.

The bar shown is obviously a homemade version. Many of these homemade pull-up bar kits can be found for free on the Internet, complete with instructions. Make sure it can support your weight and is safe!

THINGS YOU MIGHT WANT BUT DON'T NEED (AWAY)

1) GYM MEMBERSHIP

I will always remember my first visit to the gym. I looked around for three minutes, got intimidated, and left. I just remember someone breathing heavy as he walked past me. No one was mean or anything; I just got plain scared, so I ran home to my dungeon where I continued to lift weights for years. It wasn't until I started high school that I returned to that same gym, and this time I joined. That's what growth (age and muscle) can do for a kid. I was determined to go back and get huge.

I'm not going to lie, the gym is a lot of fun, but it costs a lot of money and has its dangers (usually the people there that are trying to "help" you and give you "advice"). On the other hand, you can learn a lot there, too.

The greatest danger in the gym is NOT knowing how to try an exercise suggested to you. It is extremely important that you KNOW your body enough to assess the new exercise's compatibility with YOUR body. Listen to me, listen to others, but ALWAYS make your own choice.

2) A PERSONAL TRAINER

Trainers are great, but only the BEST trainers realize how important it is for a client to understand his own body.

Be honest with yourself and answer this one question: "Why do you want a trainer?"

Some people want trainers so they can *learn*. . . .
Some people want trainers for *motivation* . . . .
Some people want a trainer for other reasons . . . .

In the end, it doesn't matter WHY you want a trainer, just as long as you're honest with YOURSELF as to why.

I DO RECOMMEND AT LEAST *ONE SESSION* WITH A QUALIFIED TRAINER IF YOU STILL ARE UNSURE OF HOW TO PERFORM THE EXERCISES.

AS A CHEAPER ALTERNATIVE (FREE), I HIGHLY RECOMMEND VIEWING VIDEOS OF THE EXERCISES IN THIS BOOK FROM A REPUTABLE WEBSITE. BE SURE TO COMPARE THIS BOOK'S EXERCISE DESCRIPTIONS WITH ANY VIDEO YOU WATCH.

"S-C-H-O-P" MOTIVATIONAL BRAIN TRIGGERS

How do you motivate yourself? This is something you are stuck figuring out on your own. It comes down to finding at least ONE way to motivate yourself.

Here are my top FIVE suggestions:

#1 SEEING

Try sticking up a picture or sign someplace where you'll see it every single day, such as on the refrigerator. What picture or message you put up is solely up to you.

#2 COPYING

People are always copying each other. It's not always cheating. Copying is a way for us to learn. This could be done by watching countless Internet videos or by watching someone perform a particular exercise in the gym. This book is another fine example of how to learn by copying.

#3 HEARING

The other motivational tool I suggest is creating a "playlist" (a collection of songs on one of many electronic devices). These songs should be played whenever you work out. Every time you hear a song on your playlist, it will remind you to workout.

#4 OTHERS

Having someone to work out with or a personal trainer helps some people maintain motivation and focus. Sometimes having an obligation or appointment will keep you consistently exercising.

#5 PHYSIQUE

Unlike some, I recommend weighing yourself each day at the same time (once-a-week at the very least!) because it will get you focused. Keep in mind it's normal for your weight to fluctuate up and down during the day. You may gain muscle and lose fat, but typically, if you start gaining weight and you look different in the mirror, this will give you motivation to eat a little healthier or work out a little more. Actually looking at your body each day is another recommendation. When you look at yourself in the mirror (whether you're muscle-posing or not), you are dealing with how your body looks and your self-image; love yourself mentally and take care of yourself physically.

DIET + MIND

"The fuel you choose to run your body."

CRAVINGS

You may not be a certified dietitian, but I know you've heard, "You are what you eat." It doesn't take a genius to know what foods and drinks are good for you and which are not. And let's face it, we all CRAVE certain foods and beverages. Our bodies seem to get addicted to certain things, too. Be very AWARE of what you crave and eat. Know your enemy, keep it close, and conquer it by creating methods to fight and win.

- For example, guzzling a glass of water can curb cravings. Eating smaller meals/snacks more often throughout the day can also help balance hunger obsessions.
- If you must, eat a TINY portion of the craving, such as ONE piece of chocolate.
- Keep yourself busy.
- "RUN!" Psychologically, if you just do something like randomly start running around your house or relocate yourself, it can change your state of mind. Not to mention it's kind of funny. The ideas and possibilities are endless.

Keep in mind that a lot of your typical cravings will disappear once you start eating REAL foods.

JUNK FOOD

Usually you hear about people craving carbohydrates or "carbs." Ignoring the fancy words for now, let's just call it all *junk food*. Junk food is stuff that is *processed* (not by YOUR body) and contains a bunch of things most people can neither pronounce nor understand. This stuff might even have addictive stuff added to it, whether it is natural or artificial. And, of course, you can read about this topic for hours on the Internet. The point is, certain foods will keep you coming back for more and in larger amounts.

SUGAR

Sugar . . . sugar . . . sugar. The average daily recommendation for grams of "table sugar" (could be listed as sugar or "high fructose corn syrup") is around *twenty-five grams per day*. This is just basically the "sugar" or "high fructose corn syrup" that food makers add to their food products. I hate using the fancy words, but you'll find a huge debate on real sugar vs. high fructose corn syrup. In the end, *twenty-five grams per day or less* of sugar is the recommendation. This isn't easy!

Some twenty-ounce drinks have around seventy grams of "sugar" or "high fructose corn syrup." That's three times the recommended amount.

I hope you see where I'm going with this. When you start looking at foods and drinks, you'll probably find out that you're consuming TONS OF SUGAR each day. Sugar can be a major craving and problem.

PILLS, POWDERS, AND MAGICAL POTIONS (AGAIN)

Here's another area you could spend months reading about. In the end, you should be able to skip all of this stuff by simply eating real food and drinking water. I really don't think there are any short cuts. The best thing you can do is actually work out. While many see supplements as an "insurance policy" for getting enough protein and/or vitamins and minerals in their diet, too much of these supplements can end up being extra calories. As mentioned before in the Four Truths section (#3), supplements are not required.

REAL FOOD

- Fruit
- Vegetables
- Nuts
- Grains
- Meats
- Beans
- Dairy

The trick with real food is that the LESS it is processed the better. It is much better for your BODY to process/digest the foods you eat. More details later . . .

WATER

The body is around 60 percent water. This is the best overall DRINK you should be consuming. I've never measured out sixty-four ounces every day, but drinking a *few* glasses of water throughout the day is probably very reasonable.

Keep in mind that for years the mantra was "Drink eight (8 oz.) glasses per day." Now and again you'll see articles stating that "sixty-four ounces of water a day is too much and unnecessary . . . and . . . and . . . and . . . could actually be bad for you."

So what's the answer? I follow the same advice both today and during my most youthful days when I was in the best shape of my life. Just keep it simple and use common sense.

Drink water when you're thirsty!

PORTIONS AND CALORIE CALCULATORS

At some point, you need to figure out how much you're eating. No matter what you eat, moderation goes a long way. Eating *smaller* meals more frequently throughout the day helps keep you from craving and overeating. It also keeps your body running steadily throughout the day.

Yes, you could eat only three *larger* meals each day, but it could lead to over-eating because you're so darn hungry by mealtime. Similarly, eating six larger meals could lead to overeating.

In the beginning, I think it is best to use a little math (counting calories) for a few days until you learn what is considered a "serving" for YOU. Remember that a 200-pound person is going to require more food than a 100-pound person.

Don't let this information cause you to panic. In the end, the mere fact that you're going to be lifting weights (building strength and muscle) will offset a lot of "mistakes" in your diet. Your body will tell you when it's hungry. It's much more difficult to "diet" when you aren't doing any exercise because when you're inactive, every single calorie seems to count more.

Don't forget that MUSCLE will burn calories twenty-four hours a day, but if you *really* want to burn calories, there's nothing like USING MUSCLE. Moving and being active is the best overall calorie burner.

You can find calorie counters all over the Internet to estimate the calories you need based on age, height, weight, and how active you are throughout each day. But as you will see, your WEIGHT and ACTIVITY LEVEL matter most. Here are some examples to give you an idea of how wide the range can be:

100-pound Male

Inactive	**1,800 calories per day**
Active	**2,500 calories per day**

200-pound Male

Inactive	**2,500 calories per day**
Active	**3,500 calories per day**

Again, how much you weigh and how much you work out are the main factors. Adjusting your calories up or down will determine whether you gain or lose weight.

RULES IN ORDER TO RULE

"Five rules that will help you stay healthy and injury-free."

LESS IS MORE (TEARING AND HEALING MUSCLE)

You may not want to never, ever take a day off from training once you start, but to lift every single day forever will actually exhaust your body and do a lot less for you, and *that's* just plain stupid. This is why "Less is More."

RULE #1

Never work out a muscle that is sore. Wait until the muscle is NOT sore for a full day. Train it the day AFTER the no-sore-day at the earliest. Note the following example:

Day 1	train chest muscle	(tearing muscle)
Day 2	chest muscle is sore	(healing)
Day 3	chest muscle is not sore	(healing, perhaps healed)
Day 4	probably safe to train the chest again	(tearing muscle again)

In some of the more advanced workouts in this book, you will notice right away that training a primary muscle again three days later is about the best possible intensity one can expect when weight training a muscle with multiple sets. (This, of course, is a naturally healing human body.)

In many cases, after a really intense workout, taking MORE rest time (and in many ways working out LESS) can lead to BIGGER, BETTER RESULTS. It sounds crazy, but the body needs to heal in order to grow.

Now, this doesn't mean you can take off as many days as you want all the time. That's just pushing it. However, many serious lifters take off very large chunks of time during certain weeks of the year in order for the body to truly rest.

SORE (NOT PAIN) IS YOUR FRIEND AND GAIN

RULE #2

Muscles should get sore sometimes. Exercises that cause pain should be modified and/or avoided.

While this may seem obvious, it is always worth mentioning. After each work-out, you may or may not get sore. Typically you'll feel a little something. Don't become obsessed with being sore for every workout. The world may tell you that being sore every time is really important. Either way, soreness should go away within a few days. The first time I trained my calf muscles (leg muscles above the ankles and below the back of the knees) really intensely, I was sore for over a week; it was scary! I thought I'd damaged them. As it turned out, I overdid it. Still, if something becomes extremely sore or painful (and it wasn't the first time you tried the exercise), you may have damaged something more than just muscle. Pain is LOSS, not gain; only soreness is your ally, friend, and GAIN.

DON'T CHANGE (WELL, NOT TOO OFTEN)

RULE #3

You do NOT need to change your program all the time. It's better to just add weight and stick with the most effective exercises.

You will hear from a lot of people that the body needs constant change to grow. This gets you to thinking that it's best to change your workout and the exercises all the time. Yeah, I'm sure there's some science behind this, and all that "What doesn't kill you, makes you stronger!"; "You gotta change it up!"; or "Keep the body guessing!" Sure, but some exercises are just a waste of time.

You know what really changes things? Weight. When you add weight to an exercise and still control it, the muscles always feel the change. So next time someone tells you to make a change and offers up some awkward exercise, just politely decline and add a few pounds to the basics.

LIFT LIGHT WEIGHTS LIKE HEAVY WEIGHTS

RULE #4

Control the weight no matter how heavy or light. Don't be in a hurry.

Always choose weights that *you* control. Your body should move and look the SAME whether you're lifting light or heavy.

SLEEP LIKE "*RIPPED* VAN WINKLE" & "*BENCH* FRANKLIN"

RULE #5

Get a lot of sleep. Possibly 8–10 hours for teenagers.

You might not get the jokes above, but let me tell you, sleep is no joke. The body's resting period is the time when your mind and body heal and grow; take your sleeping patterns seriously. Every morning when you gaze into the mirror, you'll notice how ripped you look, but don't sleep too long or you'll overdo it.

Another man of great wisdom once said this about sleep patterns: "Same time to bed, lift, and rise, makes a man grow swole with size."

BODY PARTS

"You need to know your body before you start using it."

You can spend days learning EVERY muscle in the human body, but it's better to spend your time working out and learning those details in your biology class during the human anatomy unit. Here are some basic parts with a few specific areas.

UPPER BODY
- **CHEST** "PECS" (PECTORAL)
- **BACK**
  - "TRAPS" (TRAPEZOIDS) (below the neck to the right and left)
  - UPPER BACK
  - "LATS" (LATISSIMUS DORSI) (wings/sides of your midback)
- **ARMS**
  - FOREARMS
  - BICEPS (BIS) "buys"
  - TRICEPS (TRIS) "tries"
  - SHOULDERS (DELTOIDS) "delts"

MIDSECTION (CORE)
- **STOMACH** or "ABS" (ABDOMINALS) (ABDOMEN)
- **LOWER BACK** (area just above your butt and tailbone)

LOWER BODY
- **LEGS**
  - "QUADS" (QUADRICEPS)
  - "HAMS" (HAMSTRINGS)
  - CALF muscle or CALVES

* The BODY CHARTS to follow will help you learn about your body.

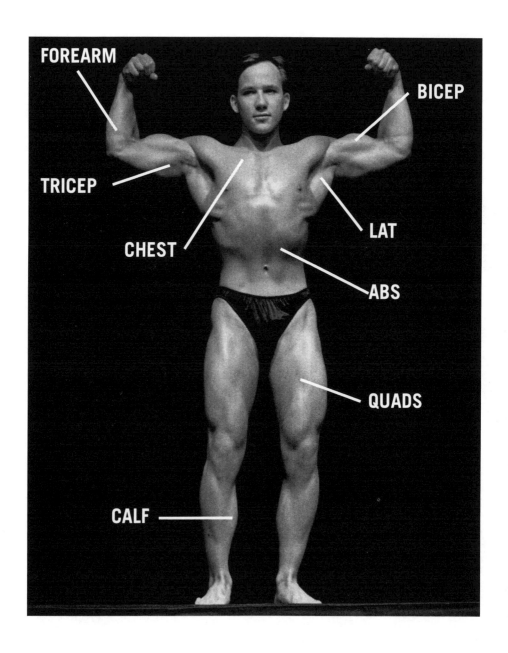

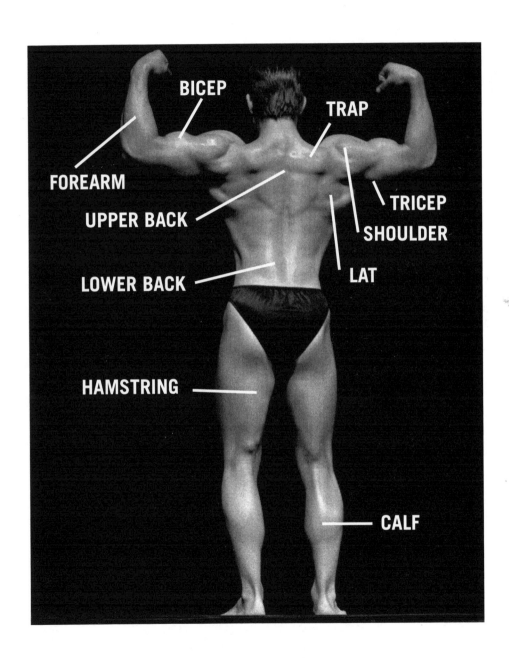

BICEP

TRAP

FOREARM

UPPER BACK

TRICEP

SHOULDER

LOWER BACK

LAT

HAMSTRING

CALF

BODY TYPES "THE BIG THREE"

We all have different bodies. Genetics dictate a lot (if not everything). Most fitness books and articles will discuss the three soma (body) types: ectomorph, endomorph, and mesomorph. Say what? These are basically categories for how the body looks. In the end, genetics, genetics, and genetics matter most. The three "types" below should be taken lightly. The idea is that you will condition YOUR body through healthy eating and training to make it look the way YOU want it to look. Researching body types is likely a waste of time. Eating properly and working out will save you from a lot of extra reading, confusion, and misdirection.

TYPE 1   "FAT" (ENDOMORPH)

This body's muscles won't be very defined due to the extra body fat covering them. This person probably eats a lot of unhealthy foods or way too many calories.

TYPE 2   "SKINNY" (ECTOMORPH)

This body's muscles show really well because of very little body fat. This person probably eats healthier foods, and either a balanced amount or a really low amount of calories.

TYPE 3   "MUSCULAR" (MESOMORPH)

This body's muscles will be well-defined and larger. This person will probably be someone who lifts weights and eats a balanced amount of calories to maintain lower body fat levels in order to look muscular and strong.

All three of these "types" can be healthy unless taken to extremes. Most people who purchase fitness books and read fitness articles are looking to lose or gain weight while building strength and muscle. Again, everyone who can lift weights can increase his or her strength and size based on genetics. Don't let someone tell you your body type is going to make things difficult for you. It's your genetics that place you into these categories based on the way you look. The way you look will not account for what kind of muscle fibers you have. You won't know until you start lifting! Will your arms get huge? Will you get super strong but lack size? Maybe you'll get a lot of both. The good news is that you WILL get SOMETHING.

BEFORE YOU LIFT

"Don't just start grabbing weights and doing random exercises."

It seems like there is a new exercise or exercise program invented every week. Most exercises are too specialized and, basically, a waste of time. All we hear about is changing your workout constantly and tricking the body all the time. Trust me, simply adding more weight does wonders, but super heavy weights can be an issue down the road. It all depends on your goals and understanding of the risks. Yes, that's right, all exercise poses a risk. The body can be damaged if you treat it like crap, so it's important that YOU are always in control.

YOU control the exercises;
the exercises don't control you.

So let's keep this simple. You've already learned the basic body parts, so now let's take a look at the BEST exercises for all these body parts. And, of course, you're welcome to spend countless hours on the Internet studying different exercises for each of the five basic body parts: chest-back-arms-legs-stomach.

Don't worry, though. I've done a little of the research for you (thirty years of training and reading) and have put together several different exercise programs for you to choose from depending on your individual goals (side effects) . . . beyond The *Real* Goal, of course.

PICKING UP WEIGHTS (MORE THAN MANNERS)

Having good gym manners or gym etiquette means picking up your weights after use, but that's NOT the point here. How to pick up weights from the rack or floor is something most people ignore. It's possible to almost instantly injure your lower back by reaching out to grab a small weight and then slightly twisting your body with even a five-pound weight. Likewise, if you pick up a heavier weight off the ground without bending your knees, you increase the chances of pulling a muscle or worse. Learn how to lift weights with your entire body by centering yourself over the weight, squatting down, and lifting with your legs, core, and arms. Never turn or twist your body while lifting the weight. Ask any doctor, the twisting of the torso/body while reaching out for a weight or holding a weight out in front of you can be deadly to your discs in your back. These are some of the reasons why people injure their back while doing simple things like gardening. The reach and twist can be the end of you. Live to lift another day.

SETS AND REPS

This is something you need to know so that you can read about and follow different workout programs. Repetitions (reps) mean how many times you lift the weight from the time you pick up the weight until you stop lifting it due to exhaustion. Ten reps means doing a push-up ten times in a row. Sets mean you intend to do a certain amount of repetitions more than once. Imagine doing ten push-ups and then you stop because you're tired. That's one set. If you rest for a minute or so, then do another ten reps, that's your second set.

My workout today will be five sets of ten push-ups. This will be a total of fifty push-ups. Typically, you won't hit ten reps for each set because your body will continue to wear out. Unless you're so strong that you can do 100 push-ups without stopping, you will probably have trouble doing ten each time for five sets. It might look something more like this: 10, 10, 8, 8, 7. This represents five sets of varying reps using the SAME weight or body weight each time.

REST PERIOD BETWEEN SETS (2–3 MINUTES)

After you complete a set, whether it's a warm-up set or a more difficult set, you need to rest for a period of time. Breathing and taking time to either walk around or sit on the bench for a moment is important to give your body the time to reenergize itself. You can find A LOT of information on this topic; however, once again, common sense goes a long way here.

If you're out of breath after a set, rushing back into a second set is probably going to result in fewer reps. Resting a little longer would have gotten you five more reps or so with the SAME weight.

For the purpose of gaining muscle, two to three minutes between challenging sets seems about right. Rushing to the next set always leads to a loss of quality in your workout. Going fast and not being well-rested will undoubtedly lead to sloppiness of form. While there are reasons to shorten your rest period, building muscle requires more recovery time.

After you complete a few workouts, you'll find out real quick how starting a set too early can result in a really crappy set (meaning only a few reps (3 or 4) when you expected to do way more (like 9 or 10).

Use your best judgment and start each set when you feel strong again. Keep in mind I don't EVER remember looking at a stopwatch or clock between sets.

Finally, during your two to three minute rest time, I recommend spending that time quietly, thinking about whatever comes to mind. Some like to visualize the next lift; however, I always found strength in thinking, dreaming big. Once you grab the weights again, narrow your focus and target the next set.

SPEED

By now you're starting to realize that even BASIC weight training requires more thought than one might think. For the most part, you want to do the exercises in a controlled way. I like it to take me about one second to lift the weight and another second to lower it. If you were to count this in your head it would go something like this, "One-One Thousand (weight lifted), Two-One Thousand (weight lowered)." Anything close to this will appear to be a well-controlled lift. This is about as fast as I would lift. Again, it's all about controlling the weight's movement. Dropping the weight down fast or attempting to swing it up quickly will simply make it easier for your muscles to do it, and you will run the risk of injuring yourself. Live to lift another day.

CHOOSING THE RIGHT WEIGHT, SETS, AND REPS

If a weight is too light, you probably won't get much out of it. If the weight is too heavy, you'll risk injury because your muscles don't have the strength to **control** it. The weight will end up controlling **you**. Once you get a weight you're comfortable with, it makes sense that the more reps and sets you do, the more your muscles are getting worked.

So . . . what's the perfect balance between **weight, sets**, and **reps** to attain strength and maximum muscle growth without overusing the body or getting injured?

The answer is in the question: you must find the perfect balance (by listening to your body and by using the proper variation in your workouts) between **weight, sets**, and **reps**.

It might help to have a specific rep number in your head prior to lifting the weight, and then depending on how many reps you actually get, you can adjust the weight accordingly, either higher or lower.

Don't worry. After a few weeks of training, YOU will be able to figure out what's right for your body.

LIGHT WEIGHT AND HIGH REPS (15–20 REPS OR MORE)
(does nothing)

If the weight you choose for an exercise is really light, you'll be able to do a lot of reps. Light weight and high reps are good for warming up before lifting heavier weights. That's it. Forget about light weight and high reps will tone you. That's nonsense for both men and women. Light weight does nothing for strength, muscle growth, and toning. Nothing. It merely moves the muscle and burns energy. Granted this is better than doing *nothing*, but you can do much better!

In fact, if you have a joint injury, sometimes high reps can cause more soreness and inflammation than doing lower reps with a heavier weight. Super high reps can wear out a joint.

HEAVY WEIGHT AND LOW REPS (6 REPS OR FEWER)
(increases strength and power)

Assuming you can control the weight, if you choose really heavy weight for an exercise, it's going to really shock your body. When you can only lift something a few times, it puts a lot of strain on the muscle and the joints. MAYBE you can go heavy ALL THE TIME when you're younger, but a workout program like this will lead to injured joints as you age. You must find a way to balance between *light-weight-high-reps* and *heavy-weight-low-reps*.

MODERATE WEIGHT AND MODERATE REPS (8–12 REPS)
(increases muscle mass)

The answer! Well, not entirely. No matter whether or not your goal is pure strength, muscle mass, or both, there has to be balance. Without balance, all roads lead to muscle pulls and injuries. If you do a program like this a long, long time and increase your weights, it will build you strength and size to wherever your genetics will take you; however, if you occasionally add some heavy weight and low rep training, you may get to your genetic plateau much quicker.

The **Huge in High School**™ workout program in this book attempts to strike the perfect balance between increasing strength and muscle mass as quickly and as safely as possible. Again, this is for those that want to take their body to its maximum. It can be a risky and tricky process. The other workouts in this book will offer healthy alternatives. In the end, if you approach weightlifting moderately, you'll be a weightlifter for the rest of your life no matter what age. Live to lift another day.

BREATHING

NEVER HOLD YOUR BREATH!!!

This is a lot more important than you might think. You need to learn how to breathe while you work out. The breathing process protects you from creating internal stress in your body (which could explode!). It also gives you strength.

You are fairly safe as long as you're BREATHING during the exercise, but learning when to breathe IN and OUT can really help you control the exercise.

Always breathe OUT while doing the "hardest" part of the lift, usually PUSH-ING or PULLING weight.

Always breathe IN while doing the "easier" part of the lift, usually LOWER-ING weight or lowering your body.

Pushing weight off your chest	=	breathe OUT
Pulling yourself UP during a Pull-up	=	breathe OUT
Lowering weight toward your chest	=	breathe IN
Lowering your body during a Pull-up	=	breathe IN

THE EXERCISES IN THIS BOOK WILL BE MARKED WITH AN "IN" AND "OUT."

PUTTING IT ALL TOGETHER

Okay, so you choose to start with a dumbbell press. Assuming that you warmed up your body a little bit by walking on a treadmill (or something like that), now it's time to warm up the specific muscle you're going to exercise. In this case, dumbbell press *mainly* works the *chest*, but it also works the *front shoulders* and *triceps*.

ANYWAY, the best way to warm up for the dumbbell press is by warming up with a LIGHTER weight. By choosing a lighter weight to do your first SET, you are helping your body avoid injury (some people may tell you to stretch the muscle, but there are many reasons NOT to stretch, so I avoid stretching until the END of my entire workout). More on stretching later.

After you do one SET of the light weight, you can choose a weight that will challenge you for a certain amount of reps, perhaps a weight you can lift ten times. As mentioned before, the next few sets you may or may not get all ten reps. Figuring out your weights takes some "trial and error" practice, AND the amount of REPS and SETS you choose controls MANY other factors such as how many days you will rest that body part. All these choices will determine what RESULTS you can expect from exercising.

Remember to breathe during the exercise.

Once you review the different workouts, you'll start to notice WHY the **weight, reps, sets**, and **how often you work out** MATTERS.

Be patient and keep reading. Give yourself some time to digest the information above. Now let's take a look at the exercises, how to do them, and what parts of the body they work BEFORE you start studying the suggested workouts provided with this book.

MUSCLE NEVER WORKS ALONE

Exercises usually work more than one muscle (but some aren't worth mentioning). This is why resting and healing time is so important. It is also why you have to watch which exercises you group together. Here's a quick, *simplified* reference chart to show you which muscles are worked with each exercise. It is split into primary (doing the most work) and secondary muscles (if worth mentioning). This information is also available in Chapter 7 Exercises.

EXERCISE	PRIMARY MUSCLES	SECONDARY
Bench Press	Chest	Front Shoulders & Triceps
Pull-ups	Back "Lats"	Rear Shoulders & Biceps
Bent-Over-Rows	Upper Back + "Lats"	Rear Shoulders & Biceps
Squats	Legs "Quads" + Butt	Hamstrings
Seated Calf Raises	Lower Calf	
Standing Calf Raises	Upper Calf	
Bicep Curls	Biceps	
Triceps Extensions	Triceps	
Lateral Shoulder Raises	Middle Shoulder	
Upper Abdominal Crunches	Abs & Core	
Lower Abdominal Crunches	Abs & Core	
Superman Lifts	Lower Back & Core	
Planks	Abs & Core	
Side Planks	Side Abs "Obliques" & Core	
External Rotator Cuff	Shoulder "Core Muscles"	
Internal Rotator Cuff	Shoulder "Core Muscles"	

TRAINING THE SAME MUSCLES TWO DAYS IN A ROW

It doesn't make sense to train the same muscles two days in a row, especially when doing multiple exercises with multiple sets and reps. This can happen in some workout configurations, so you have to make sure there is enough rest time afterward. As a teenager, you can get away with it a little bit. In the **Huge in High School**™ workout program, the overlap on Day 3 and Day 4 was only possible due to youthfulness. As you age, you will want to insert more resting periods. This will make more sense once you look at the different workouts.

EXERCISES

7.

> **"Here are some basic exercises, what they build, and how to do them properly."**

In the pages to follow are pictures and descriptions of the MAIN exercises. I tried to stick with exercises that balance safety, risk, and cost; but don't worry, some of the mass-building variations will be included in the actual workouts chapter (10. SAMPLE WORKOUTS). Some of the simpler exercises like push-ups don't have pictures, and some of the difficult, higher-risk exercises don't, either. These will, however, be discussed so that you can determine whether you want to try them or not.

The techniques to follow make a lot more sense as you start to challenge your body with heavier and heavier weights.

*Please note which body parts and muscles (simplified) get trained as shown in parentheses below the exercise name.

DUMBBELL BENCH PRESS
(Chest + Front Shoulders & Triceps) *

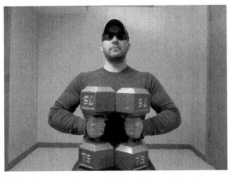

Start with the dumbbells in a safe position, resting on your legs.

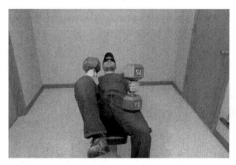

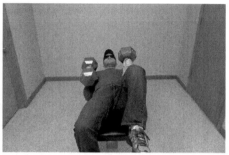

Lean back on the bench while bringing one leg up at a time to help lift the weight to the starting position. This takes tremendous strain off your shoulders all while strengthening the muscles that balance the weight. This is MUCH different than just lifting a bar off a rack or using a machine.

Now kick up the second leg to get the second dumbbell into the starting position. Notice the other leg is down for stability. This process emphasizes safety and balance.

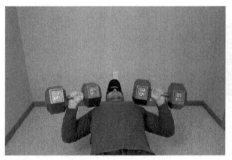

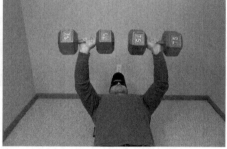

Now you're in the starting position. It doesn't have to look pretty. The main idea is that you're well-balanced on the bench and you're supporting the weight. As soon as you feel balanced, it's best to begin pressing the weight up.

As you press the weight up (breathe OUT), be sure to STOP BEFORE your elbows "lock out." This should be the highest position you go to when pressing up. (You may notice that your natural position on the bench has your head, upper back, and butt touching the bench. Your lower back is NOT.)

In a controlled manner, slowly bring the weight down (breathe IN) to the starting position.

PULL-UPS
(Back "Lats" + Rear Shoulders & Biceps)

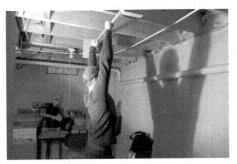 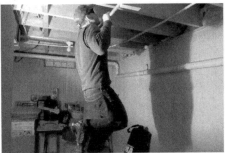

Hang from a pull-up bar so that your feet are off the ground, palms facing forward.

Pull yourself up (breathe OUT) until the bar is below your chin near your chest. No need to touch the bar to your chest or put your chin over the bar! Stay away. You don't want to smack your chin on the way back down (breathe IN). If you can't do ONE pull-up, you will have to get assistance from a partner or a machine such as a "Lat Pull-down" machine. Please also consider substituting pull-ups with the "Lat Pull-down" machine if you're over forty years of age.

ONE-ARM BENT-OVER-ROW
(Upper Back + "Lats" + Rear Shoulders & Biceps)

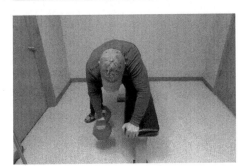

Pick up a dumbbell from the ground. The other arm and leg will be centered on the bench. During the exercise, you will NOT touch the dumbbell to the floor until the set is finished.

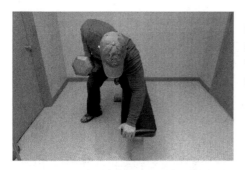

Pull the dumbbell up toward the side of your chest (breathe OUT). Lower the weight (breathe IN) being careful not to rest it on the floor and then repeat.

DUMBBELL SQUATS—LIGHT WEIGHT TRAINING ONLY

(Legs "Quads" + Butt & Hamstrings)

This is a relatively "simple" way to learn about a squat. It is **dangerous** to do heavy weight using this method. You can't hold heavy weights and properly concentrate on the FORM of your squat at the same time.

For more intense workouts, you will require a squat rack, barbell, and a whole lot of practice. I always suggest watching a lot of videos and having an experienced trainer take a look at your form. Nowadays you can even film yourself to examine where your knees, back, and feet are while you do the lift.

There is also much debate about how deep you should squat. I think it really depends on your body and perhaps your age (youthful bodies can be more forgiving). Your knees, flexibility, and lower back (and the list goes on . . .) determine the outcome. Probably the safest for your back and knees would be stopping around chair height or "parallel." Some choose to squat just below parallel and some squat down even further, pretty much down to the floor. This is NOT with dumbbells, of course.

This is an amazing exercise for your body, but it isn't something you just haphazardly do. PLEASE start with light weights and learn the FORM that works with your body. Sometimes due to flexibility issues, people can't squat properly, so they're better off starting with a leg press machine.

Typically, everyone can squat without weight and with proper form by holding onto something in front of him like a secure basement post. Again, this would be performed using just your body, no weights.

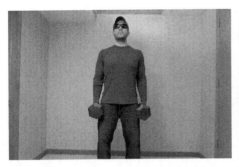

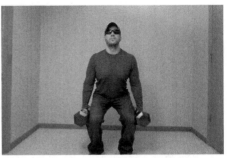

Hold two dumbbells at your sides. Be sure not to let the weight pull your shoulders down. Hold the weight up, keeping your shoulders in their natural position.

Slowly squat down (breathe IN). Knees should be above and lined up with your toes as if you can draw a straight line from your knee to your toes. The dumbbells should feel like they are a part of your body. This is much different from having a heavy bar on your back.

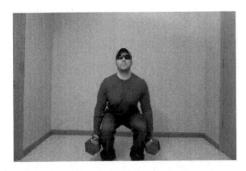

Stop around the height where you would be sitting on a chair. Then push back up (breathe OUT) to the starting position. Going too low can result in an injury to your lower back!

PLEASE REFER TO THE "SQUATS AND DEADLIFTS" SECTION

SEATED/STANDING CALF RAISES

(Lower Calf & Upper Calf)

Standing Calf Raises not shown

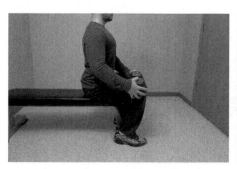 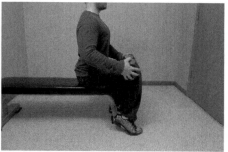

Rest a dumbbell above your knee (place it on a pillow or pad for heavier weight). You can also stand the dumbbell upright, resting one end on your leg (this will require that you balance it, though). At this point, your foot is flat on the ground as if you were standing.

Raise your foot up on its toes (breathe OUT).

Then lower your heel to the ground (breathe IN).

Repeat.

If you want to increase your range of motion (how much you move your calf up and down), you can place a small board under your toes/front of your foot. This will allow your heel to drop below your toes during the lowering movement.

The "STANDING CALF RAISE" can be done with weights (such as just holding two dumbbells at your sides) or without weights simply by raising yourself up and down on your toes. A stair step can be used to increase the range of motion during the lowering movement as well. Instead of weights you could also consider doing this exercise with ONE leg at a time, essentially doubling the weight.

DUMBBELL BICEP CURL

(Biceps)

Hold dumbbells to your sides, thumbs forward.

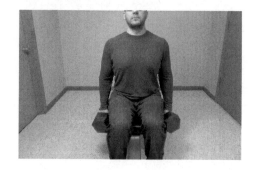

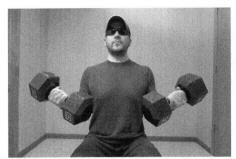 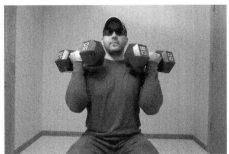

Naturally begin to lift (curl) your arms up while keeping your elbows at your sides. Don't press your elbows to your sides. Just let your body naturally curl the weight up. As you pass your legs, let your hands/palms face up toward the ceiling (breathe OUT). This movement should happen naturally so that the dumbbells move slowly toward the top of the movement.

Notice at the top of the movement the dumbbells and hands are in a position impossible to do with a barbell. This is another example of how dumbbells allow your body to move where it's most natural. Lower the weight (breathe IN) and allow the thumbs to rotate up again so the dumbbell can lower without hitting your legs. Repeat the movement. (If the rotating of your hands is driving you crazy, feel free to position your legs close together; however, this is typically uncomfortable for males.)

DUMBBELL ONE-ARM TRICEPS EXTENSION
(Triceps)

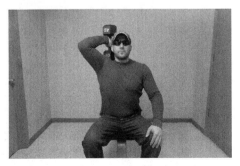

Using one or two hands, get one dumbbell positioned behind your head, resting on your upper back (on the trapezoid muscle). Now you should be able to rest it comfortably there and balance it with one hand.

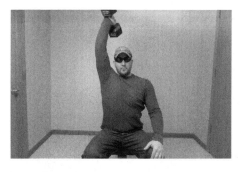

Begin to raise the weight up toward the ceiling (breathe OUT). Do not straighten your arm or "lock out" your elbow. Keep it slightly bent. Like every joint in the body, this will keep balance, keep tension on the muscle, and keep tension off the elbow joint. Lower the weight (breathe IN) being careful NOT to rest or bounce it on your back again until you've completed all the reps. This is NOT a push. Keep your elbow in the same relative position, just in front of your head. Again, controlled, slower movements are a must for this exercise. All the power should come from your triceps muscle.

SIDE LATERAL SHOULDER RAISES
(Middle Shoulder)

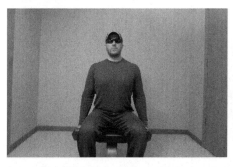 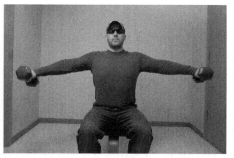

Start with your hands at your sides, thumbs pointing forward. Your hand position will not change as it did in the bicep curl. Raise the dumbbells up and out away from each side of your body like flapping wings (breathe OUT).

It is best to STAY BELOW "parallel" with the floor or where your arms are perfectly straight out. Lower the weight (breathe IN). Repeat. (Elbows remain in a "locked" position, which is okay because the weight isn't pressing the joints together.) Heavy weight can be very dangerous due to high pressure on the shoulder joint/rotator cuff muscles. It has also been suggested that it is SAFER to turn your thumbs toward the ceiling a little bit or all the way. Never "pour the can" or tip the dumbbell so that it faces the floor. This can lead to a shoulder strain/pinch/impingement.

There are versions of this exercise that allow the elbows to be bent, which allows for heavier weight. Your choice, but it can get dangerous. Another option that exists is where you KEEP your thumbs rotated UP as you raise the weight up. Also, your arms will be slightly in front of your body rather than directly to your sides, almost as if you were attempting to hug a giant ball. It may help to look up "Lateral Dumbbell Raise in the Scapular Plane." Currently, this is considered the safest method for a lateral raise.

UPPER ABDOMINAL CRUNCHES

(Abs & Core)

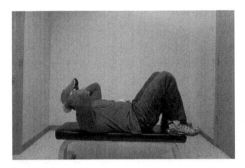

Slowly crunch upward, bringing your shoulders and upper back up off the bench a little bit (breathe OUT). Then lower yourself back flat to the starting position (breathe IN). This exercise can be simple as long as you're not pulling on your head and neck. You're resting your head in your hands (fingers locked), keeping your chin OFF your chest. You shouldn't feel any tension in the neck. You have to learn how to use ONLY your abdominal muscles to crunch or sit up a few inches off the bench. There are MANY variations of this exercise.

LOWER ABDOMINAL CRUNCHES "TOES TO CEILING HIP RAISE"

(Abs & Core)

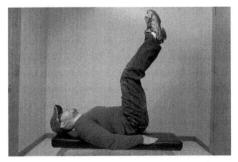

Lie flat on your back with your legs pointed up. Lift your butt and part of your lower back off the bench (breathe OUT). Then lower your back and butt down flat on the bench again (breathe IN). Repeat. The picture shows the END position where the lower back and butt are off the bench. This is a very short movement. It is NOT the same as a leg lift where your legs start near the floor and then raise up.

* The BICYCLE CRUNCH EXERCISE is considered the most ADVANCED and EFFECTIVE movement that combines BOTH the Upper and Lower Abdominal Crunch. This is an exercise you want to look up to understand the movement once you are comfortable with the basic crunch exercises. *

** Upper and Lower Abdominal Crunches have been said NOT to work the core muscles as deeply as exercises such as Planks; and more recently, it has been suggested that major power movements such as SQUATS and DEADLIFTS are the true strengtheners of the body's deep CORE. **

*** Traditional Sit-ups (coming all the way up) are considered dangerous to your neck, back, and spine. Sit-ups can lead to herniated discs, compressed vertebrae, and nerve damage. ***

SUPERMAN LIFTS
(Lower Back & Core)

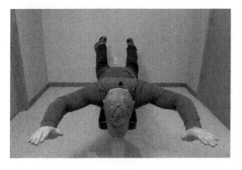

This core exercise is a one-position (isometric) "movement," meaning your body will stay still and tense as if you were holding a pose. Lie flat on your stomach while holding out your arms and legs as if flying. You should feel pressure and muscle tension from your butt through all of your back to your shoulders. Hold this position for 60 seconds. Build up to this amount of time. Breathing will be normal throughout this exercise. (You may want to explore whether or not longer time intervals create diminishing returns, meaning it may not strengthen the area any more after so many seconds.)

PLANKS
(Abs & Core)

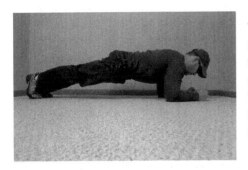

This is another isometric (one-position) exercise. Hold yourself above the floor while only your toes, elbows, forearms, and fists touch the floor. Keep your body in a relatively straight position. Breathe normally while holding for a goal of 60 seconds.

SIDE PLANKS
(Side Abs "Obliques" & Core)

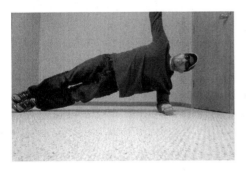

Start off this isometric movement by lying on your side, flat on the ground. Stack your feet and lift yourself into position by balancing on one elbow, forearm, and fist. Point your opposite arm toward the ceiling/sky, forming a "T" shape. Pressure and tension will be felt in your side abdominal muscles (obliques) closest to the floor/ground. Breathe normally while holding for a goal of sixty seconds. Repeat on the other side, of course!

EXTERNAL ROTATOR CUFF

(Shoulder "Core Muscles")

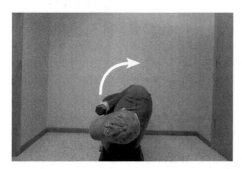

Lie flat on a bench. This exercise is NOT about how much weight you can use. Ten pounds goes a long way, while most people start with five pounds. Take a light weight dumbbell and while placing your arm against your side, rotate your arm up and out like a door swinging open. Your elbow is your door hinge. Your forearm should be the only part of your body moving. Note the arrow in the drawing above. This is typically a ten to fifteen rep exercise. If you feel a kind of burning in the shoulder joint, that usually means you've done enough. No need for any extreme intensity while doing this movement. This movement is performed in a slow and controlled manner.

This exercise is primarily for strengthening, stabilizing, and protecting your shoulder joint from imbalance due to heavy lifting or an imbalance in your larger muscles as you weight train. (It is recommended that you look up information on the rotator cuff's anatomy and purpose). Many believe the *external* rotator cuff exercise guards BEST against an imbalance in the shoulder due to heavy chest and back dominance training (which leads to the overstrengthening of the shoulder's *internal* rotational power.)

It is EXTREMELY important that you do NOT LIFT ANYTHING over your head or do any HIGH-SPEED movements with your shoulders such as throwing a ball or swinging a bat/racket AFTER ANY multiple-set rotator cuff training.

INTERNAL ROTATOR CUFF
(Shoulder "Core Muscles")

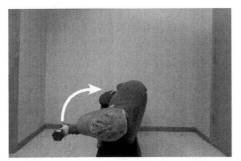

Same position as the external rotator cuff movement, except you use the opposite hand to rotate up toward your chest. Please note the arrow. All the same restrictions apply to this exercise as the external rotator cuff exercise.

Keep in mind that both the external and internal rotator cuff exercise can be done while standing up using "Bands" of resistance tied to a door knob or something on the wall. The "Bands" are just what they sound like, thick rubber bands designed for exercise, especially used in the rehabilitation of the shoulder when it's injured.

There are MANY variations and exercises that build different parts of the rotator cuff. While it's possible that some people don't do these types of movements at all, I feel that these inner-strength exercises have protected my shoulders from imbalance and harm. Please take the time to learn about the four rotator cuff muscles "SITS": Subscapularis, Infraspinatus, Teres minor, and Supraspinatus.

Live to lift another day.

KNOW THYSELF

"Know what you want, the risks and rewards."

Strength comes from the inside (core), inner strength. Weight training and exercise helps build and connect your inner and outer power. Bodybuilding exercises can be different from power lifting exercises. A traditional bodybuilder vs. a power lifter (strongman) can have very different looking bodies. It's, after all, very much up to you which path you choose and/or a combination of the two. Just imagine the workout program and diet of a Japanese Sumo wrestler!

Power lifting is said to come from Squats, Deadlifts, and the Bench Press where faster speed, lower reps (between one and six), and heavy weight are the key to accomplishing its main goal: strength and power. Some swear that the workout below does it all:

Squat	1.5	x	your body weight
Deadlift	2.0	x	your body weight
Bench Press	1.5	x	your body weight

Power Cleans are also an interesting exercise for building explosiveness in sports, but these concepts will be discussed briefly in section **11. FINAL WORDS** under the heading "Sports Specific Training."

Bodybuilding, its main goal being increased muscle mass, is said to come from moderate reps (between eight and twelve), slower movements, and variable weight. Bodybuilding also focuses on using many more exercises both general and specific to the body's muscle groups.

The real question is whether or not you care about all those inner, HIDDEN muscles. You may have noticed that the last five exercises (Superman Lifts, Planks, Side Planks, External Rotator Cuff, and Internal Rotator Cuff) may seem a little pointless. After all, you won't really see these areas bulge through your shirt or even skin for the most part. So why waste your time?

The reason rests in creating a strong core by strengthening the surrounding stabilizing muscles in your entire body, in order to protect your joints. Damage to your body's internal and hidden parts will turn your body into a pile of weakened mush.

Again, if you're focusing on The *Real* Goal then it makes sense to focus on some sort of middle ground between both power lifting and bodybuilding so as to maintain your maximum health and strength throughout your entire lifetime.

RISKS AND BENEFITS OF CERTAIN EXERCISES

Now that you've learned a bit about the body and its movements, it is time to revisit the risks and benefits of certain exercises. For the most part, whenever your arms are positioned OVER your head or ABOVE your shoulders, it places your shoulder joints in very stressful positions, depending on the exercise. Pushing/Lifting weight over your head places a higher risk of strain on your shoulders. You won't find any over-the-head **shoulder presses** in this book. Working the *front* of the shoulder is risky (and usually gets overdeveloped) and requires a lot of knowledge on form. If you decided to add this exercise, plan on treating it like the squat and deadlift. A person can get enough secondary front shoulder training by doing the **Dumbbell** (or barbell) **Bench Press**.

Pull-ups are a bit different. They work a very large area of your *back* as well as *biceps* and the rear of the *shoulder*. That being said, there are a ton of factors regarding the strain on your shoulders: height, weight, upper body strength, age, etc. This exercise is not as complicated to do as the **Squat**; however, it would be beneficial to have a trainer take a look at your form. A GREAT alternative to this exercise (much lower risk) is the "Lat" Pull-down machine (pulling the bar down as if you're doing a pull-up, but **never** behind the head). The financial downside is that you'll need to buy one or join a gym. (Please review "Push-ups and **Pull-ups** Beyond Age Forty?" in section 1. INTRODUCTION)

Please remember that **Squats** (deadlifts, pull-ups, and even overhead shoulder presses) require a lot of practice and knowledge of your body as well as proper FORM and technique.

JOINTS—LIGHT WEIGHT VS. HEAVY WEIGHT

You don't want to mess up your joints: **knees, shoulders, elbows, wrists, ankles**, not to mention all the **vertebrae** along your neck and back. Many other areas exist: such as the tendon running through the bottom of your feet and the four rotator cuff muscles/tendons inside your shoulder. YOU WILL BE SHOCKED how WEAK and DISABLED your body can become if you injure any of these areas.

Constantly using HEAVY weights will eventually win the battle against your joints. Even LIGHT weight at an extremely high number of "burning" reps will overuse these areas.

The key is to train somewhere in between these two extremes and to take great caution when using HEAVY weights. WARMING-UP, FORM, REST, and paying close attention to your BODY'S ability to CONTROL the exercise will minimize risk.

"DON'T GET *CARRIED* AWAY"—THE DEADLIFT AND SQUAT

Squats

By this point in the book, a lot has been said about the SQUAT. This is yet another reminder of how the squat should be in a book by itself. This isn't supposed to be a scare tactic, but a serious reminder that as you increase the weight for this exercise (barbell only, of course, because we would never go heavy with dumbbells on this exercise), you need to increase your knowledge as well. Consider watching several professional videos as well as finding a trainer to help you learn this exercise. ALWAYS REMEMBER, however, that no matter what you read or what you are told, YOUR BODY is still your BEST COACH, so LISTEN TO IT.

Deadlifts

Here is an exercise that has NEVER been mentioned at length. This has been done ON PURPOSE so it forces you to seek out more information. The DEAD-LIFT appears to be really easy at first, but like the squat, form is extremely important, especially when you start slapping on more weight. This exercise is performed by picking up a BARBELL (NO dumbbells here, seriously) off the ground and then setting it down again. It appears to be very simple:

Place your feet flat beneath the bar. Squat down and grab the bar about shoulder width or slightly wider with your palms facing your legs (overhand grip). Lift the barbell by extending hips and knees to fully **stand up straight**. Shoulders should be pulled back at top of lift if they are rounded forward. Return the bar to the ground the same way you came up and repeat. You can also modify your grip by having ONE hand's palm facing forward (reverse grip) while the other hand is an overhand grip.

This may sound easy, but there are different hand grips and LOTS of other ways to do it wrong. There are also possible variations in the way you breathe during this exercise. Like any exercise, you can load on too much weight, break form, and injure yourself. This is an exercise that has been said to destroy your back (spine), and it is a movement that has been said to strengthen your entire body as well as protect your back (spine). Obviously it is an exercise that you have to try for yourself. I, personally, got ALL my results WITHOUT deadlifts; however, had I done deadlifts as intensely as squats, I may have gotten much better gains (or more injuries!) in my younger years. I'll never know. All I can say is that my back is in good shape, and if I do start doing deadlifts someday, I would probably keep things on the "lighter side" (eight to twelve rep weight) vs. lower rep maximums.

Squats and Deadlifts

These are two power exercises worth learning and considering. In the end, there is no question that these are two amazing exercises that build the body's size and strength. Reading about all the benefits of the deadlift makes me feel like I've been missing something all these years, but YOU can choose to do one, none, or both of these power exercises. Also consider that if you're controlling the weight and aren't going too heavy, odds are you'll maintain better form and won't get injured and still get some benefits. GOOD FORM with weight you can CONTROL always means fewer injuries (if any at all) and less chance of getting carried away on a stretcher! Live to lift another day.

JUDGE ME

My high school experience did NOT include deadlifting, shrugs (for the trapezoid muscle), or any core work other than abdominals (and squats for core) to create my physique as shown in this book. Who knows what adding them would've done. Nevertheless, these exercises have value. Remember that each of us is on our own individual journey in order to decipher the riddle of iron.

Below is a snapshot of the exercises I did most frequently to get huge in high school. You will notice right away that I used FREE WEIGHTS whenever possible.

BARBELL FLAT BENCH PRESS
BARBELL INCLINE BENCH PRESS
DUMBBELL FLAT BENCH PRESS
DUMBBELL INCLINE BENCH PRESS
BODYWEIGHT PULL-UPS
LAT PULLDOWN (MACHINE)
BARBELL BENT-OVER-ROW
DUMBBELL ONE-ARM BENT-OVER-ROW
BARBELL SQUATS
LEG PRESS (MACHINE)
LYING LEG CURLS (MACHINE)
STANDING CALF RAISES (MACHINE and BODYWEIGHT)
BARBELL STANDING BICEP CURLS
DUMBBELL SEATED BICEP CURLS

BARBELL OVERHEAD TRICEPS EXTENSION (CURL BAR)
TRICEPS PUSHDOWN (CABLE MACHINE)
DUMBBELL LATERAL SHOULDER RAISES
BODYWEIGHT ABDOMINAL EXERCISES
DUMBBELL ROTATOR CUFF EXERCISES

ADD INTENSITY
ADD LOTS OF SETS
ADD RARELY MISSING A WORKOUT
ADD EATING REAL FOOD
ADD SLEEP

NOTE ON LEG EXTENSIONS

Although a lot of lifters do these, there is now much discussion on how these are probably better for rehabilitation of the knee (when you can't put direct pressure on the joint such as after a knee surgery). I never went too heavy on these. This is why I removed them from the **Huge in High School™** *workout program.*

9.

DIETS

"There's no mystery here: you are what you eat."

You can read thousands of articles on what to eat and what not to eat, but sometimes it's best to put book learning aside and spend your time working out. In this section, you will find the basic food plan I was on throughout high school. It shows you what eating reasonably healthy can do when added to serious, consistent workouts. Here's a great example: today Greek yogurt replaces regular yogurt because it contains more protein, but "back-in-the-day" I only really knew about the regular stuff; yet miraculously, I still gained muscle. If you really want the "perfect" eating plan, then go to an experienced dietician; however, it probably isn't necessary. Eat BIG. Lift BIG. Be BIG.

WHAT TO EAT AND DRINK

Okay, let's make this easy. Drink water, tea, or coffee without sugar. Have some milk or a little bit of dairy each day. Avoid sugar-infested drinks. Eat protein, whole grains, vegetables, fruits, and healthy oils like olive oil or other healthier oils such as coconut oil. Eating a variety of foods is probably really smart. Did I mention to try to avoid sugar? You want to eat FRESH (organic is always nice), unprocessed food free of pesticides, chemicals, etc.

Here are some tough words you'll want to learn:

protein   (meat, dairy, beans or eggs)
carbohydrates (fruits, rice, breads and grains, starchy vegetables and sugars)
fats   (fish, walnuts and vegetable-based oils, nuts, seeds, avocado)
               (high-fat meats and full-fat dairy)

water   (found in drinking water)

vitamins   (found in food)
minerals   (found in food)

And, of course, you're going to find that, in the world, food tends to be an ongoing argument. To drink dairy or not . . . too much soy or not . . . all whole grains or too many whole grains . . . fat or nonfat . . . take multivitamins or don't take multivitamins . . . and on and on. Even the United States government changed its Food Pyramid!

Again, you can spend days on the Internet looking up every diet imaginable, but really it isn't that difficult.

Just eat a variety from these groups, limit junk-food, and drink water instead of sugar-based drinks. Done.

ALCOHOL "TO DRINK OR NOT TO DRINK?"

Don't drink it! You're in high school! If you're NOT in high school and of legal age, I'd say limiting this to once-a-week (hopefully not a binge) is acceptable. Again, there is a lot of back-and-forth science on this. The less you drink (if at all), the better, but as always, feel free to read all about alcohol's influence on the body in your spare time.

HUGE IN HIGH SCHOOL™ SCHEDULE, DIET, AND WORKOUTS

The following diet is what I ate in high school. This doesn't mean it's perfect by any means; in fact, it can be improved quite a bit! The point of including it here is to demonstrate the effectiveness of healthy eating when paired with an intense, consistent workout plan.

And just as a side note, if you're a finicky eater, with some discipline, you can become accustomed to eating almost anything. Simply force yourself to eat the food over and over again; eventually, you get used to eating a lot of foods without loads of added sugar. Plain Greek yogurt is an excellent example.

Diet
+
Workout
=
Your Physique

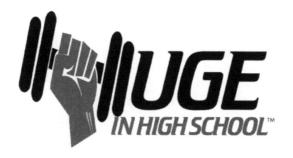

SCHEDULE

"Eat BIG. Lift BIG. Be BIG."

6 - MEALS PER DAY (365-DAY ROTATION)

(Requires WILL POWER)

MEAL #1 – Breakfast

MEAL #2 – Between Breakfast/Lunch

MEAL #3 – Lunch

MEAL #4 – After School

SLEEP (1 hour)

WORKOUT (1–1.5 hours)

HOMEWORK (1–3 hours)

MEAL #5 – Dinner

MEAL #6 – After-Dinner Snack

SLEEP (8–9 hours)

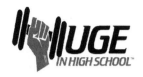

DIET AND SCHEDULE

"Eat BIG. Lift BIG. Be BIG."

MEAL #1 – Breakfast

- water or skim milk (*no milk as an adult, just water*)*
- vanilla or lemon yogurt (*plain* 0 percent *Greek yogurt today!*)*
- small can of white albacore tuna (*Wild Pacific/Alaska Sockeye/Pink Salmon today!*)*
- one hardboiled egg
- one-half grapefruit
- oat cereal or instant oatmeal (*Steel cut oatmeal today!*)*

MEAL #2 – Between Breakfast/Lunch

- water
- ham or turkey (processed meats) on wheat bread (*Unprocessed meats today!*)*

MEAL #3 – Lunch

- salad with vinegar and oil or a small amount of ranch dressing
- vanilla or lemon yogurt (*plain* 0 percent *Greek yogurt today!*)*
- skim milk (*no milk as an adult, just water*)*
- apple
- two slices of pizza and a soda pop ONE time during school week (instead of above)

MEAL #4 – After School

- peanut butter and jelly sandwich or on ten crackers or so
- skim milk (*no milk as an adult, just water*)*

SLEEP (1 hour)
WORKOUT (1–1.5 hours)
HOMEWORK (1–3 hours on/off until bedtime)

MEAL #5 – Dinner

- skinless chicken, pork chops, or steak, but sometimes just pasta, bread, and/or potatoes
- skim milk (*no milk as an adult, just water*)*
- variety of vegetables
- mixed greens salad

MEAL #6 – After Dinner Snack

- low salt wheat cracker snacks
- water

* denotes significant present-day changes/substitutions in my diet such as increased protein, lowered sugar, (avoidance of) high mercury levels in fish, and slower-burning carbohydrates.

MEAL #1 - BREAKFAST

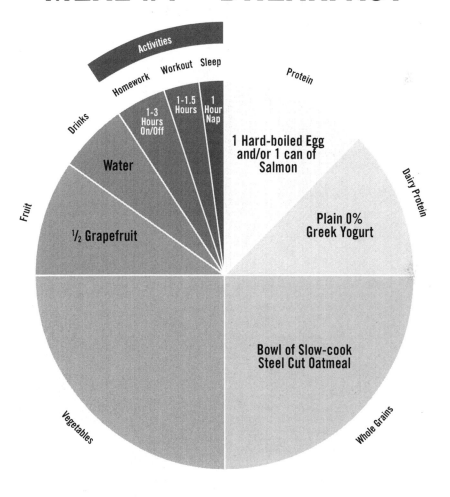

MEAL #2 - BETWEEN BREAKFAST AND LUNCH

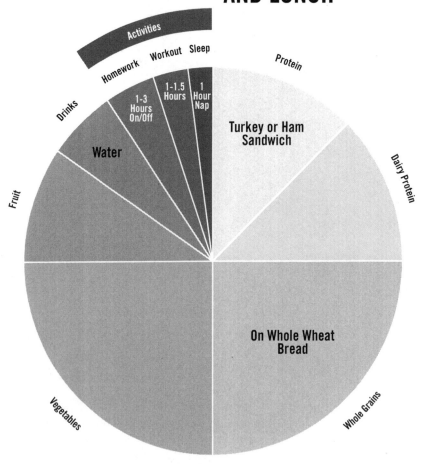

MEAL #3 - LUNCH

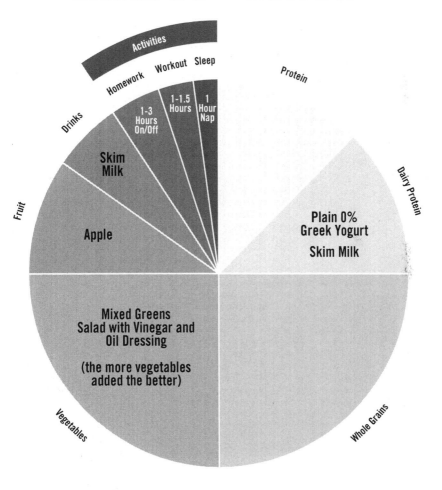

* ONE time per week you may substitute everything
above for two slices of pizza and a soda pop.

MEAL #4 - AFTER SCHOOL

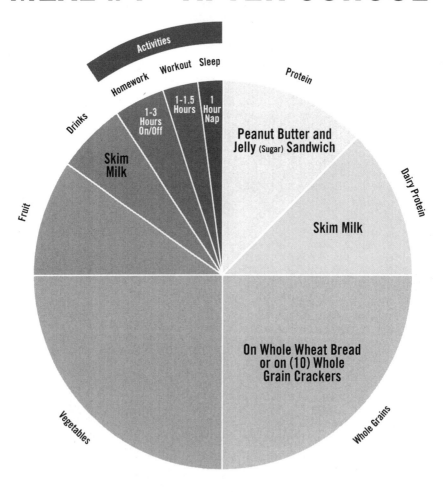

MEAL #5 - DINNER

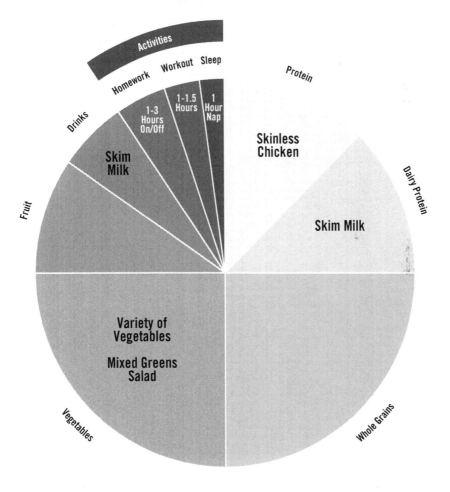

Activities

Homework   Workout   Sleep

Protein

Drinks

1-3 Hours On/Off

1-1.5 Hours

1 Hour Nap

Skim Milk

Skinless Chicken

Fruit

Dairy Protein

Skim Milk

Variety of Vegetables

Mixed Greens Salad

Whole Grains

Vegetables

MEAL #6 – AFTER-DINNER SNACK

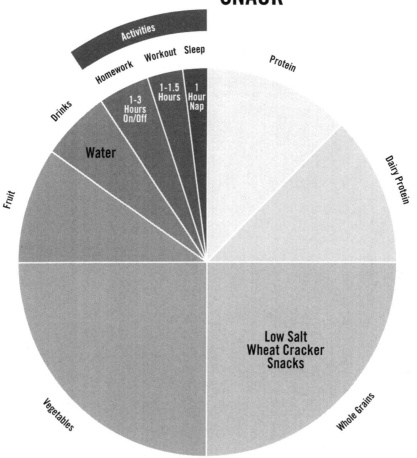

Activities

Homework   Workout   Sleep

Drinks

1-3 Hours On/Off   1-1.5 Hours   1 Hour Nap

Water

Protein

Fruit

Dairy Protein

Vegetables

Low Salt Wheat Cracker Snacks

Whole Grains

24-HOUR ACTIVITY CHART

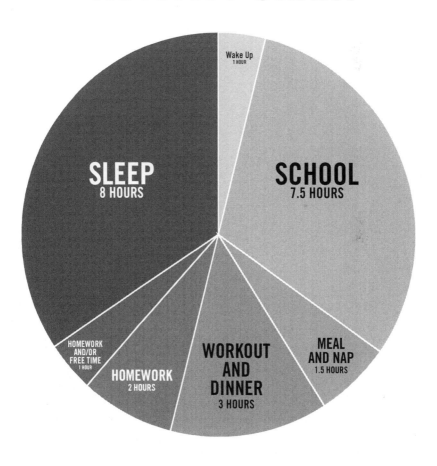

Wake Up
1 HOUR

SLEEP
8 HOURS

SCHOOL
7.5 HOURS

HOMEWORK
AND/OR
FREE TIME
1 HOUR

HOMEWORK
2 HOURS

WORKOUT
AND
DINNER
3 HOURS

MEAL
AND NAP
1.5 HOURS

WORKOUTS

"Choose wisely."

Just in case you skipped or skimmed chapters 1–9 and jumped right to the workouts, at least consider this: before you blindly follow one of these programs (besides clearing it with a physician first), make sure you start out slow. In fact, you can cut down on the sets while you figure out what amount of weight is good for you on each exercise. It will take a few weeks to adjust to the overall strain on your entire body. Take your time so you don't get injured or too sore to lift for a week! It can happen! Once you condition your body, you'll be ready to ramp up the intensity each week.

THE "MAX" FACTOR *OLD*

As long as you're moving your body around in life, you'll probably remain reasonably healthy. There are so many different types of activities and exercises you can do. It's probably important to realize that plenty of people just WALK their whole lives and live well into their eighties and nineties.

I once had the honor of training a man named MAX who had NEVER really worked out in his life. Max had just come out of a short-term coma (yes, coma) from an apparent collapse while playing golf (yes, golf). Once he was released from the hospital and had been home a few days, he drove HIMSELF over to the gym and signed up to work with a personal trainer (me). The conversation went something like this:

(ME)   "Hi, Max. Nice to meet you, so what type of exercising have you done all your life? Have you ever lifted weights before?"

(MAX)   "Oh, I just walked."

I was in my twenties at the time, and he was **ninety years old!**

THE "MAX" FACTOR *YOUNG*

In my thirties, as a school teacher, I had the absolute honor of teaching a young man named Max. We kept in touch after he graduated from high school and then something unexpected happened. Max passed away; he was only twenty years old. At 6'5" and 220 pounds, he was everything you would expect from a young man involved in physical fitness. The autopsy revealed Max died of *an enlarged heart*. This type of tragedy might have been avoided by having what's called a "Healthy Heart Check." This requires both an echocardiogram (ECHO) and an electrocardiogram (EKG). These are simple and painless tests and well worth your time. ALWAYS clear any workout plan with your doctor BEFORE starting a program.

INTENSITY AND RISK

It is important that YOU decide exactly where you want to start. While there are risks everywhere in life, it is still important to consider your point of focus and tolerance of risk factors. Exercise does NOT have to be an extreme activity, depending on your overall goals. Here are some simple guidelines.

BASIC HEALTH   "I-just-want-to-be-in-shape."

This program would probably consist of a lot of low-impact moving such as walking attached to a very relaxing weight training program. If not weights, then probably body weight exercises and general calisthenics.

LOW-RISK HUGE   "I-want-to-push-my-body-and-build-as-much-muscle-as-my-body-can-while-still-training-as-safely-as-possible."

This exercise plan would definitely require some form of weightlifting with moderately heavy weights, fewer sets, around the ten rep range.

HIGH-RISK HUGE   "I-want-to-push-my-body-and-build-as-much-muscle-as-my-body-can-while-still-training-as-safely-as-possible-with-the-heaviest-weights-possible-at-times."

*This high-intensity plan would require weightlifting with heavy weights and a plan similar to the **Huge in High School**™ workout program.*

IT'S TIME TO PICK A WORKOUT

The following workouts are based on doing multiple sets of each exercise. This is why it's important to have proper resting (healing) periods. The **Huge in High School**™ workout program, **7-DAY VARIABLE WORKOUT (14-DAY ROTATION),** is most likely the maximum for any teenager (or natural human being). This is an ADVANCED program. Each body part is trained twice per week with only one complete day of resting. Despite having done this workout as a teenager, you should eventually move toward a training frequency that allows for more resting time. EVERY workout listed after the **Huge in High School**™ workout program is *easier* and allows for more healing time, or they can serve as BEGINNER programs.

<u>Let your body decide which workout best fits you when you start and as you age.</u>

The 8-Day and 10-Day workouts create more healing time after the entire body has been trained, which is accomplished in three days (thus the fancy term "3-Day Split" because you train the entire body in three days). Of course, there seem to be endless variations such as the "4-Day Split," etc. As long as you follow the general principles, pretty much any variation you create will be effective.

(SAMPLE)

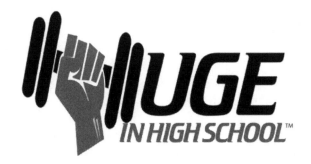

WORKOUT PROGRAM

"Eat BIG. Lift BIG. Be BIG."

(HIGH-RISK HUGE)

7-DAY VARIABLE WORKOUT (14-DAY ROTATION)

(Requires a GYM or a lot of home equipment)

Day 1	(Monday)	Chest/Back
Day 2	(Tuesday)	Legs
Day 3	(Wednesday)	Arms/Shoulders
Day 4	(Thursday)	Chest/Back
Day 5	(Friday)	Legs
Day 6	(Saturday)	Arms/Shoulders
Day 7	(Sunday)	OFF

⚡*HUGE* WORKOUT VERSION "A" ⚡*HUGE*

DAY 1 (MONDAY) CHEST & BACK

Body Warm-up (slow) • **5–10 minutes** • **(treadmill, bike, etc.)**

(Sets do NOT include a low-weight warm-up set)

Barbell Bench Press	5 sets	8–12 reps	225 lbs. (Choose your
Barbell Incline Bench Press	5 sets	8–12 reps	185 lbs. own weight.)
Pull-ups (50 reps)	5 sets	8–15 reps	body weight only
Barbell Bent-Over-Row	5 sets	8–12 reps	185 lbs.

*Core Work (Abdominal exercises, planks, etc.)
*Rotator Cuff exercises (2–3 sets) (Perhaps with a focus on external cuff muscles.)
*Light Stretching
*Intensity and reps vary from day-to-day based on soreness, etc. Use common sense and listen to your body.

DAY 2 (TUESDAY) LEGS

Body Warm-up (slow) • **5–10 minutes** • **(treadmill, bike, etc.)**

(Sets do NOT include a low-weight warm-up set)

Squats	5 sets	8–12 reps	225 lbs.
Leg Press	5 sets	8–12 reps	405 lbs.
Leg Curls	5 sets	8–12 reps	100 lbs.
Standing Calf Raises	5 sets	20 reps	300 lbs.

*Core Work (Abdominal exercises, planks, etc.)
*Light Stretching
*Intensity and reps vary from day-to-day based on soreness, etc. Use common sense and listen to your body.

DAY 3 (WEDNESDAY) ARMS & SHOULDERS

Body Warm-up (slow) • **5–10 minutes** • **(treadmill, bike, etc.)**

(Sets do NOT include a low-weight warm-up set)

Barbell Bicep Curls	4 sets	8–12 reps	115 lbs. (standing)
Seated Bicep Curls	4 sets	8–12 reps	50 lbs. (dumbbells)
Overhead Triceps Extension	4 sets	8–12 reps	115 lbs. (curl bar)
Triceps Pushdown	4 sets	8–12 reps	110 lbs. (machine)
Side Lateral Shoulder Raises	5 sets	8–12 reps	30 lbs. (dumbbells)

*Core Work (Abdominal exercises, planks, etc.)
*Rotator Cuff exercises (2–3 sets) (Perhaps with a focus on external cuff muscles.)
*Light Stretching
*Intensity and reps vary from day-to-day based on soreness, etc. Use common sense and listen to
  your body.

⫸HUGE WORKOUT VERSION "B" ⫸HUGE

DAY 4 (THURSDAY) CHEST & BACK

Body Warm-up (slow) • 5–10 minutes • (treadmill, bike, etc.)

(Sets do NOT include a low-weight warm-up set)

Dumbbell Bench Press	5 sets	8–12 reps	90 lbs. (dumbbells)
Dumbbell Incline Bench Press	5 sets	8–12 reps	75 lbs. (dumbbells)
Pull-ups (50 reps)	5 sets	8–15 reps	body weight only
Dumbbell Bent-Over-Row	5 sets	8–12 reps	90 lbs. (dumbbells)

*Core Work (Abdominal exercises, planks, etc.)
*Rotator Cuff exercises (2–3 sets) (Perhaps with a focus on external cuff muscles.)
*Light Stretching
*Intensity and reps vary from day-to-day based on soreness, etc. Use common sense and listen to
  your body.

DAY 5 (FRIDAY) LEGS

Body Warm-up (slow) • 5–10 minutes • (treadmill, bike, etc.)

(Sets do NOT include a low-weight warm-up set)

Squats	5 sets	8–12 reps	225 lbs.
Leg Press	5 sets	8–12 reps	405 lbs.
Leg Curls	5 sets	8–12 reps	100 lbs.
Seated Calf Raises	5 sets	20 reps	200 lbs.

*Core Work (Abdominal exercises, planks, etc.)
*Light Stretching
*Intensity and reps vary from day-to-day based on soreness, etc. Use common sense and listen to
  your body.

DAY 6 (SATURDAY) ARMS & SHOULDERS

Body Warm-up (slow) • 5–10 minutes • (treadmill, bike, etc.)

(Sets do NOT include a low-weight warm-up set)

Barbell Bicep Curls	4 sets	8–12 reps	115 lbs. (standing)

Seated Bicep Curls	4 sets	8–12 reps	50 lbs.	(dumbbells)
One-Arm Triceps Extension	4 sets	8–12 reps	50 lbs.	(dumbbell)
Triceps Pushdown	4 sets	8–12 reps	110 lbs.	(machine)
Side Lateral Shoulder Raises	5 sets	8–12 reps	30 lbs.	(dumbbells)

Core Work (Abdominal exercises, planks, etc.)
Rotator Cuff exercises (2–3 sets) (Perhaps with a focus on external cuff muscles.)
Light Stretching
Intensity and reps vary from day-to-day based on soreness, etc. Use common sense and listen to your body.

Day 7 (Sunday) OFF

⅊UGE WORKOUT VERSION "C" ⅊UGE
(WITH PYRAMIDING)

DAY 8 (MONDAY) CHEST & BACK
Body Warm-up (slow)   •   5–10 minutes   •   (treadmill, bike, etc.)

(Low-weight warm-up INCLUDED in 1st set)

Barbell Bench Press	1st set	15 reps	135 lbs.	
	2nd set	8–10 reps	225 lbs.	
	3rd set	4–6 reps	275 lbs.	(The 4th set
	4th set	4–6 reps	295 lbs.	depends on
	4th set	4–6 reps	275 lbs.	your level
	4th set	8–10 reps	225 lbs.	of strength
	5th set	8–10 reps	225 lbs.	that day.)
	6th set	8–15 reps	185 lbs.	
Barbell Incline Bench Press	1st set	15 reps	135 lbs.	
	2nd set	8–10 reps	185 lbs.	
	3rd set	4–6 reps	225 lbs.	
	4th set	4–6 reps	225 lbs.	
	5th set	8–10 reps	185 lbs.	
	6th set	8–15 reps	135 lbs.	
Lat Pulldown Machine	1st set	15 reps	90 lbs.	

	2nd set	8–10 reps	150 lbs.
	3rd set	4–6 reps	180 lbs.
	4th set	4–6 reps	180 lbs.
	5th set	8–10 reps	150 lbs.
	6th set	8–15 reps	90 lbs.
Barbell Bent-Over-Row	1st set	15 reps	95 lbs.
	2nd set	8–10 reps	135 lbs.
	3rd set	4–6 reps	185 lbs.
	4th set	4–6 reps	185 lbs.
	5th set	8–10 reps	135 lbs.
	6th set	8–15 reps	95 lbs.

*Core Work (Abdominal exercises, planks, etc.)
*Rotator Cuff exercises (2–3rd sets) (Perhaps with a focus on external cuff muscles.)
*Light Stretching
*Intensity and reps vary from day-to-day based on soreness, etc. Use common sense and listen to
  your body.

WORKOUT VERSION "C" (WITH PYRAMIDING)

DAY 9 (TUESDAY) LEGS

Body Warm-up (slow)   •   5–10 minutes   •   (treadmill, bike, etc.)

(Low-weight warm-up INCLUDED in 1st set)

Squats	1st set	15 reps	135 lbs.
	2nd set	8–10 reps	225 lbs.
	3rd set	4–6 reps	275 lbs.
	4th set	4–6 reps	315 lbs.
	5th set	8–10 reps	225 lbs.
Leg Press	5 sets	8–12 reps	405 lbs.
Leg Curls	5 sets	8–12 reps	100 lbs.
Standing Calf Raises	5 sets	20 reps	300 lbs.

*Core Work (Abdominal exercises, planks, etc.)
*Light Stretching
*Intensity and reps vary from day-to-day based on soreness, etc. Use common sense and listen to
  your body.

☠HUGE WORKOUT VERSION "C" ☠HUGE
(WITH PYRAMIDING)

DAY 10 (WEDNESDAY) ARMS & SHOULDERS

Body Warm-up (slow)   •   5–10 minutes   •   (treadmill, bike, etc.)

(Low-weight warm-up INCLUDED in 1st set)

Barbell Bicep Curls	1st set	15 reps	95 lbs.	(standing)
	2nd set	8–10 reps	115 lbs.	
	3rd set	4–6 reps	135 lbs.	
	4th set	8–10 reps	115 lbs.	
Seated Bicep Curls	4 sets	8–12 reps	50 lbs.	(dumbbells)
Overhead Triceps Extension	1st set	15 reps	95 lbs.	(curl bar)
	2nd set	8–10 reps	115 lbs.	
	3rd set	4–6 reps	135 lbs.	
	4th set	8–10 reps	115 lbs.	
Triceps Pushdown	4 sets	8–12 reps	110 lbs.	(machine)
Side Lateral Shoulder Raises	5 sets	8–12 reps	30 lbs.	(dumbbells)

*Core Work (Abdominal exercises, planks, etc.)
*Rotator Cuff exercises (2–3 sets) (Perhaps with a focus on external cuff muscles.)
*Light Stretching
*Intensity and reps vary from day-to-day based on soreness, etc. Use common sense and listen to your body.

Day 11 (Thursday) Chest/Back (RESTART with Workout A)

Day 12 (Friday) Legs (RESTART with Workout A)

Day 13 (Saturday) Arms/Shoulders (RESTART with Workout A)

Day 14 (Sunday) OFF

8-DAY WORKOUT

(Teenager & Twenties)

Day 1	Chest/Back
Day 2	Legs
Day 3	Arms/Shoulders
Day 4	OFF
Day 5	Chest/Back
Day 6	Legs
Day 7	Arms/Shoulders
Day 8	OFF

10-DAY WORKOUT

(Thirties & Beyond)

Day 1	Chest/Back
Day 2	Legs
Day 3	Arms/Shoulders
Day 4	OFF
Day 5	OFF
Day 6	Chest/Back
Day 7	Legs
Day 8	Arms/Shoulders
Day 9	OFF
Day 10	OFF

The following workouts are identical to the previous programs; however, they have a different combination of body parts. This is a preference. However, consider that these combinations allow for more rest because the secondary muscles do NOT get trained two days in-a-row as they do during Day 3 and Day 4 in the **Huge in High School**™ 7-DAY VARIABLE WORKOUT (14-DAY ROTATION) workout program.

7-DAY WORKOUT

(different body part combinations)

Day 1	(Monday)	Chest/Triceps
Day 2	(Tuesday)	Back/Biceps/Shoulders
Day 3	(Wednesday)	Legs
Day 4	(Thursday)	Chest/Triceps
Day 5	(Friday)	Back/Biceps/Shoulders
Day 6	(Saturday)	Legs
Day 7	(Sunday)	OFF

8-DAY WORKOUT

(different body part combinations)

Day 1	Chest/Triceps
Day 2	Legs
Day 3	Back/Biceps/Shoulders
Day 4	OFF
Day 5	Chest/Triceps
Day 6	Legs
Day 7	Back/Biceps/Shoulders
Day 8	OFF

10-DAY WORKOUT

(different body part combinations)

Day 1	Chest/Triceps
Day 2	Legs
Day 3	Back/Biceps/Shoulders
Day 4	OFF
Day 5	OFF
Day 6	Chest/Triceps
Day 7	Legs
Day 8	Back/Biceps/Shoulders
Day 9	OFF
Day 10	OFF

TRAINING THE BODY ONCE-A-WEEK

The next series of workouts trains the body LESS frequently. These workout plans may especially benefit those who PLAY SPORTS. For example, you would lift Monday-Thursday so as to leave healing time before Friday and Saturday game days.

These workouts split the body into four or more days ("4-Day Split"), thus training the entire body only one time per week, a great way to grow and stay in shape for life at any age. Again, this type of workout would be best if you want to make your training life a bit easier.

In theory you could do double the sets (twenty sets for larger body parts), but tearing the muscle down to nothing and needing longer heal times seems a bit counterproductive and a great way to get injured.

If you're really looking to pack on the maximum amount of muscle, then you should train the body closer to two times per week with a reasonable number of sets as shown in the 7-, 8-, and 10-Day workouts. (Again, NOT twenty sets for chest, but more like ten sets twice a week).

(LOW-RISK HUGE)
7-DAY WORKOUT

DAY 1	MONDAY	CHEST
DAY 2	TUESDAY	BACK
DAY 3	WEDNESDAY	LEGS
DAY 4	THURSDAY	ARMS + SHOULDERS
DAY 5	FRIDAY	OFF
DAY 6	SATURDAY	OFF
DAY 7	SUNDAY	OFF

HUGE IN HIGH SCHOOL™ BEGINNER PROGRAM

If you're just starting to lift weights for the first time, this is a great program to START with. Of course, you can modify any program on your own, but this plan starts off with fewer exercises and sets so you can do it all at home. Sometimes the gym can be intimidating, overwhelming, and downright inconvenient, but if you've read this book, you should be more than ready for anything.

The exercise plan below can all be done at home with only a little bit of equipment: **flat bench**, some **dumbbells**, and an **optional pull-up bar** (depending on your strength, age, and overall performance level.)

The PICTURES for this workout are all in **Chapter 7 EXERCISES**.

(BEGINNER)
HUGE IN HIGH SCHOOL™

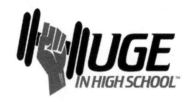

WORKOUT PROGRAM

DAY 1	CHEST + BACK
DAY 2	LEGS
DAY 3	ARMS + SHOULDERS
DAY 4	OFF
DAY 5	OFF
DAY 6	RESTART

🏋️*UGE* DAY 1 CHEST & BACK 🏋️*UGE*

Body Warm-up (slow) • 5–10 minutes • (Running In Place?)

(Sets do NOT include a low-weight warm-up set)

Dumbbell Bench Press	5 sets	8–12 reps	_____ lbs.
Pull-ups (20 reps)	2 sets	8–15 reps	body weight only
Dumbbell Bent-Over-Row	3 sets	8–12 reps	_____ lbs.

(If you are NOT doing pull-ups, do 5 sets of the One-Arm Bent-Over-Rows)

*Core Work (Abdominal exercises, planks, etc.)
*Rotator Cuff exercises (2–3 sets) (Perhaps with a focus on external cuff muscles.)
*Light Stretching
*Intensity and reps vary from day-to-day based on soreness, etc. Use common sense and listen to your body.

🏋️*UGE* DAY 2 LEGS 🏋️*UGE*

Body Warm-up (slow) • 5–10 minutes • (Jumping Jacks?)

(Sets do NOT include a low-weight warm-up set)

Dumbbell Squats (light weight only)	5 sets	8–12 reps	_____ lbs.
Seated Calf Raises	5 sets	20 reps	_____ lbs.

(You could mix these five sets with a few sets of standing raises on a stair-step using body weight or with dumbbells in your hand.)

*Core Work (Abdominal exercises, planks, etc.)
*Light Stretching
*Intensity and reps vary from day-to-day based on soreness, etc. Use common sense and listen to your body.

🏋️*UGE* DAY 3 ARMS & SHOULDERS 🏋️*UGE*

Body Warm-up (slow) • 5–10 minutes • (A Quick Walk?)

(Sets do NOT include a low-weight warm-up set)

Seated Dumbbell Bicep Curl	5 sets	8–12 reps	_____ lbs.
Dumbbell One-Arm Triceps Extension	5 sets	8–12 reps	_____ lbs.
Dumbbell Side Lateral Shoulder Raises	5 sets	8–12 reps	_____ lbs.

*Core Work (Abdominal exercises, planks, etc.)
*Rotator Cuff exercises (2–3 sets) (Perhaps with a focus on external cuff muscles.)
*Light Stretching
*Intensity and reps vary from day-to-day based on soreness, etc. Use common sense and listen to your body.

Day 4 OFF (Could ADD an activity from the "Training the Body for Basic Health" list)

Day 5 OFF (Could ADD an activity from the "Training the Body for Basic Health" list)

Day 6 RESTART PROGRAM

ENDLESS COMBINATIONS

This is yet another body part combination. For those of you who are training each body part once-a-week, here is yet another option.

DAY 1	LEGS
DAY 2	CHEST
DAY 3	BACK
DAY 4	OFF
DAY 5	SHOULDERS
DAY 6	ARMS
DAY 7	OFF

TRAINING THE BODY FOR BASIC HEALTH

The list below is an example of some of the healthy activities you can ADD to any of the fitness programs. Usually these activities would be performed on days when you're not lifting weights.

STRETCHING	YOGA	DANCING	SPARRING
WALKING	HIKING	BOUNCING	JUMPING ROPE
SPORTS	RUNNING	SWIMMING	CALISTHENICS
BIKING	SPRINTING	AEROBICS	KAYAKING

CARDIOVASCULAR "CARDIO" TRAINING

I rarely did any traditional cardio as a teenager such as running a mile. I simply kept active by walking, hiking trails, and doing activities instead of sitting all day. (This doesn't count as cardio (or does it?), but I definitely trained an hour a day with heavy weights).

UNLESS you're training for a particularly high-energy, extreme sport or preparing to run a marathon, cardiovascular training doesn't have to be as grueling as some make it out to be. Remember, ninety-year-old Max "Just Walked."

Ideally cardio should be performed eight to twelve hours apart from weight training or on nonweight-training days. Do cardio after weight training if done together. Cardiovascular training is a book in itself if you're into marathons and similar events, but remember that anything extreme comes with higher risk.

Using cardio training strategically, as noted above, can definitely help you burn body fat. Just be sure you aren't overdoing it, and remember to eat enough healthy foods. You don't want your calorie count to become too low. (Don't forget that you're working out all the time.)

Consider being active throughout the week and you'll find that the body fat will slowly start to go away.

STRETCHING I

Kind of like the "How much water should I drink per day?" debate, stretching is similarly packed with fact and myth. If you can keep your body *reasonably flexible* throughout your life, you'll be perfectly fine. Typically, a warm-up such as treadmill or exercise bike is sufficient before lifting weights; however, many times I found myself briefly stretching my legs and chest before the warm-up set. Again, never for a very long period of time and certainly nothing extreme like the splits before squats! (No way!) In fact, I only remember stretching my chest and legs for about a minute or so before doing the bench press or squat. The most stretching took place during my squat workout if I felt too tight or cramped.

Modern ideas claim that doing a warm-up set is the most important and effective way to protect and prepare a muscle for heavier lifts. Now I don't feel so bad doing five-minute warm-ups on the treadmill and then jumping right into the bench press as a teenager . . . but I always did a warm-up set.

The latest research seems to suggest that stretching a few times a week AFTER any type of exercise is considered a good idea. Here are some areas worth stretching if you want to relieve some of the body's tension: hips, hamstrings, calves, and back.

Here's what I did as a TEENAGER and now as an ADULT:

- Five- to ten-minute warm-up on treadmill or stationary bike. (Keep in mind you could simply run in place or do jumping jacks. Just move around and warm the body a bit.) One could argue you don't have to do this at all, just so long as you do a warm-up set for the muscle you're about to train; however, I'm in favor of a quick warm-up, anyway. It can't hurt!
- Briefly stretch the chest (before a chest workout) and legs (before a leg workout). If my legs weren't feeling good after my first warm-up squat, then I would typically stretch the calves, hamstrings, and quadriceps. (Remember, there are strong arguments *against* stretching before a lift or even a run!) This idea revolves around loosening up the muscles and joints when they're supposed to remain tight for strenuous lifts or runs in order to do their job: keep stuff together and in alignment.

I say go by the feel of your muscles before and after the warm-up set. If the muscle doesn't feel right, do another warm-up set. Often times I found myself doing an extra light set of squats because my legs or knees felt stiff. On rare occasions, after two light sets and some stretching, if my legs and knees still felt tense (or my lower back didn't feel right), I would simply go home. Better to "skip leg day" than end up with major damage in your joints or spinal discs. When something doesn't feel right, don't do it. Live to lift another day.

STRETCHING II

It is important that you LEARN how to stretch all the main body parts. You can find this information anywhere with easy-to-follow pictures. Use common sense. Don't go insane and try to stretch too far or do the splits (unless, of course, you're training to do the splits).

Taking a day or two out of the week (or whenever you're feeling tenseness in your muscles) to stretch is probably best. This means just stretching for the heck of it. Many people feel and build tension in their hips, lower back, and legs. You would be surprised how little aches can miraculously disappear after you stretch and loosen the tightness in the hips.

The trick is to remember to TAKE YOUR TIME and BREATHE. Let stretching in itself be a *RELAXING* activity. Don't be in a hurry. Slowly move into the stretch and hold it for awhile. Nothing quick and don't bounce up-and-down or back-and-forth. Above all, stick with stretches that FEEL GOOD. No crazy neck stretches or extreme body positions. Here are the main areas to focus on:

CHEST

SHOULDERS

QUADRICEPS

HAMSTRINGS

CALVES

HIPS

YOGA (slow-flow or gentle) is an excellent class to sign up for to learn all about stretching. Keep it safe, comfortable, and don't do anything extreme.

FINAL WORDS

"Hey, Bro . . . "

As this book comes to its end, it is important to list information on the seemingly endless topics that come up whenever one talks about exercise. This section of the book is the place to empty out all the advice I have left (or that I remember), everything from my collective learned experience.

The greatest and sometimes most dangerous thing about learning to work out is getting advice from others, both solicited ("Hey, Bro. What do you do for arms?") and unsolicited ("Bro, you're doin' that wrong.")

Here are three "doings" that will MESS you up when going the natural way and thinking long term:

1. doing too much
2. doing it wrong
3. doing drugs

Remember what you've learned from this book and you shouldn't run into too many issues differentiating between good advice and bad advice. In the end, if you listen to YOUR body, it'll guide you.

TO BUY OR NOT TO BUY

Isn't that always the question in fitness?

Since the 1960s, fitness books, special programs, fancy equipment, and, of course, "secrets" have been selling . . . selling . . . and selling strong to this very day. I'm not sure this now $1 billion industry will ever come to an end. Yes, I'm

WELL AWARE you've purchased this book with your hard-earned money, and that's why I'm suggesting that you continue to spend *wisely* on the *exact* things *you* want.

It takes WORK to increase your muscle and strength. It also takes COMMON SENSE, BALANCE, and REASON to stay healthy. Please continue to have safe, long-term goals; and please continue to purchase things you will actually use, such as a stable weight bench or perhaps an excellent personal trainer instead of "crazy and amazing" programs or "do-it-all" equipment. And if you do decide to purchase something from the Land of Gimmicks, please make sure you TEST it against the principles and concepts in this book. Remember, almost ANY MOVEMENT will help you get in shape; however, it takes a steady, controlled, and consistent program to build muscle and strength. Only then will you reach your maximum genetic self.

The ONLY way this process will become irrelevant or wrong will be due to a MIRACLE drug that helps you safely grow muscle and strength without doing anything. Yes, that's right. I mean you will be able to just sit around and not work out at all. Just swallow a pill, inject something, or drink some magical or scientific potion of power and you, too, will gain muscle and strength. But even then your MIND will know you did NOTHING to get the muscle and strength. Hmmm, that *might* bother you.

Nevertheless, nothing like this currently exists, anyway.

WEIGHT BELTS, KNEE WRAPS, AND GLOVES

Do you need any of this stuff? The short answer is "NO!"

WEIGHT BELTS

If you are going to be a professional power lifter or strongman, then the weight belt will become important for one rep max-outs during competitions. Other than crazy heavy lifts (typically 85 percent of your max or higher), it is probably best to never use a belt. By the way, if you do use a belt, you should know how to wear one. Things such as belt placement and tightness matter. The best thing

I remember about my weight belt was it had my name in big letters across it. Eventually I stopped using it. Relying on a weight belt can actually weaken your core. Again, it's your choice. If you're getting really advanced and using really heavy weight on extreme lifts such as squats and deadlifts, then a belt is probably a good idea for extra protection during your gargantuan, heavy sets.

KNEE WRAPS

The same goes for knee wraps as it does for weight belts: use only in extreme cases. Arguably, these would really just be for extreme lifts by extreme power lifters. I used them a few times, but then I got worried about weakening my knees. No thank you. Then again, my personal best was four reps at 315 lbs. down to the ground (way below parallel) after my regular squat workout. No wraps. Fortunately, that event got me thinking about just how much weight was I willing to do before my knees would break. If you're not a competitive power lifter, maybe it's best to set certain limitations for the long haul. Live to lift another day.

GLOVES

Gloves are going to protect your hands and should increase your grip, but unless you have sweaty hands, the gloveless hand works just fine. Some of you will enjoy the feel of the cold iron. You can always wash your hands after your workout. Expect to get calluses just under your fingers on the palm of your hand. Some see these as marks and rough spots to be proud of. Gloves or no gloves, it's your choice.

SPOTTING

Let's consider the Barbell Bench Press. Sometimes when you're lifting (and you're young), you may want to go those extra reps (forced reps) or you may just want to protect yourself from dropping a barbell on your chest. Asking for a spot from a workout partner, a gym employee/trainer, or a club member (a stranger?) requires attention. Make sure you set up a CLEAR communication system between yourself and the spotter. One word commands, such as "up" work great.

Also be sure your spotter knows what do to once you say "up" or "help." I believe it's best to have the spotter keep the weight MOVING at all times. Even during this forced rep, the body keeps moving, which is a lot safer than stopping, failing, dropping the weight back down to your chest, and THEN having a spotter help you lift it off. Remember, you can have three spotters on a bench press; however, this would probably only be necessary for an extremely heavy lift (a one rep Max-out, which I do not recommend).

FORCED REPS

If you're going to force out extra reps with a spotter, it is probably best done when you are *young*. AFTER you have already done as many reps as your muscles can take and have fatigued (tired out), your spotter helps you do a few more repetitions (forced reps) of an exercise by assisting you with the weight. Again, it is important that the spotter keeps the weight moving. This way the lifter can maintain proper form. You can perform these when you are in your forties, but the risk of joint issues goes up. Better to stop when your muscles are tired. Live to lift another day.

CHEAT REPS

These are pretty obvious. Cheat reps are kind of like a semi-risky way to spot yourself. For example, if you are barbell or dumbbell curling, you could start to rock or lean your body backward to help jerk the weight up a bit in a "controlled" manner. I recall doing this VERY carefully with heavier barbell bicep curls; however, for the sake of your back, you are probably better off with an intelligent spotter.

ONE REP MAX-OUTS

As fun as this can be, it is a bad idea. Unless you are a competitive power lifter, there is probably no good reason to "max-out" on any exercise with ONE extreme rep. Yes, I did it, but it also took its toll on my joints. This can be permanent damage. At age eighteen, weighing 171 pounds, I maxed 300 pounds on the bench press. It may sound great, but it was foolish. If you already know you can lift 275 for six reps and 295 for four reps on a really strong day, then why take the chance to max-out? Common sense would tell you that you could hit 300. Eventually the weights will increase during your workouts and when 300 pounds is in the rotation, you will know you can max over 300, maybe even 315. In this case, it is safer to *know* rather than to prove. Live to lift another day.

STRIP SETS

Like forced reps, strip sets attempt to accomplish the same thing: exhaust the muscle. With strip sets you lift a weight as many reps as you can and then quickly lower the weight for an immediate second set, lower the weight again, third set, and so on. Sometimes called a "burn-out" set, you can continue to do this for five sets, ten sets, as long as you can go until you completely "burn" or "fry" the muscle. Obviously this will promote (maybe guarantee) soreness for the next day. I did not do these very often unless I was really bored or in a hurry to get a workout finished. I also don't like the idea of getting really sloppy with your form. It can get a little crazy. Live to lift another day.

PYRAMID SETS

Pyramid sets or "pyramiding" is just what the name implies. You start with a lighter weighted set, and then add weight for the next set until you reach your heaviest weight. Then you lower the weight for each set. If you like math, and you graph the sets and numbers, it would form a pyramid on a graph. A version of this type of training shows up in the **Huge in High School**™ Workout Program (Version "C").

SUPERSETS

Lots of weightlifters like to really make things interesting and start "flying" all over the gym doing one exercise after another. I do remember trying a superset going between two different exercises for different body parts: biceps and triceps

- One set of Barbell *Bicep* Curls . . . then immediately after (no rest)
- One set of Overhead *Triceps* Extensions (curl bar).

For a natural weightlifter, this probably isn't necessary. Again, it can lead to sloppy and out-of-breath sets, and imagine if you decided to superset two exercises that work the SAME muscle. This just ends up being a kind of STRIP SET, exhausting the muscle.

Overall, you rarely need to play these "games" in the gym; you can steadily grow by ADDING WEIGHT to exercises while maintaining CONTROL of the weight. You want intensity? Add some resistance and force yourself to get those reps!

SPORTS-SPECIFIC TRAINING

If you are playing a sport in school, it is important to first realize that aggressively lifting weights during the season could actually lower your performance. Be sure there is plenty of time for full recovery of your muscles before a game. You don't want to hit the field with sore or even fatigued muscles.

Sports-specific training explores the idea that you can train in a certain way to enhance your performance in a certain sport. Typically exercises implementing **plyometrics** (explosive movements such as jumping) may increase your vertical jump in basketball or your acceleration when running. The Power Clean is said to increase explosive strength, but it is an extremely advanced movement. Some say deadlifts and squats will build power more safely than Power Cleans. Sports training can get complicated, but does it have to be?

Athletes should consider copying professional workouts used by professional sports teams or seek out advice from a professional athlete in your sport of choice.

Most likely, a combination of sport-specific movements and weight training will be the best way to increase your performance.

You won't see a professional male basketball player bench pressing super heavy. His shoulders are required to make shot after shot, not lift a two-hundred pound basketball.

The connection between weightlifting and your particular sport can get very complicated. It is important to really know your goals so you do not damage a joint or muscle, risking loss of playing time, or worse, getting knocked out for the season.

Above all, watch out for nonsensical workouts or gimmicks that have unrealistic claims.

ADVICE FROM SOMEONE ELSE'S SKULL

I remember guys in the gym that swore by an exercise called "Skull-crushers" for triceps. You lie flat on your back, on a bench, with a curl bar fully extended above your body in the bench press position. You then slowly lower it toward your forehead (skull) in a similar arc as in most triceps exercises, bending at the elbows. I tried this exercise once and it KILLED (pain and discomfort) my elbows. This was with virtually no weight on the curl bar. For some reason it placed my elbow joints in an awkward position, again, pain doing the movement with just the curl bar (no added weight) . . .

. . . but when doing an Overhead Triceps Extension using a curl bar (similar to the Dumbbell One-Arm Triceps Extension on page 59), I could lift 135 pounds for reps! Had I tried that heavy on Skull-crushers, not only would I have trashed my elbows, but I would have, well, crushed my skull. Pay attention to your body. Live to lift another day.

POSTURE

This may seem foolish, but how you walk about, stand, and sit in a chair is extremely important. Rather than go on-and-on about this, it's probably best to just remember to "Stand up straight!" and "Sit up straight!" Be conscious of how your back is positioned. If you sit and walk around and you feel like you're tired and slouching your back, most likely your posture is wrong. Incorrect sitting or standing positions will usually lead to stiffness or irritation of the neck and back. The good news is that, with proper weight training, you will naturally become more and more aware of good form and posture as you increase your weights in each exercise.

When discussing posture and form, this would be a good time to remind you that the more weight you use on an exercise, the more your body's structural flaws are at risk (or may reveal themselves due to the stress). This is why slowly growing your strength and controlling the weights and the exercises are so important.

THREE STRANGE INJURIES AND THEIR SOLUTIONS

Let's face it, we all get overenthusiastic at times and overdo it. Sometimes injuries are accidents or just plain mistakes. Either way, MOST injuries heal quickly and only set back your workouts a week or so, but what about STRANGE injuries? These injuries can reoccur if you don't know their origin.

This is where a little obsessive-compulsiveness comes in handy. These injuries may not occur with everyone, but they are still worth mentioning. More than one weightlifter has dealt with some of these issues, but who knows, you may not.

#1 THE HAND MUSCLE PULL

That's right! You can pull a muscle in your hand. Having used many different types of dumbbells, I found that, as you get into the heavier ones, the handle really starts to matter. Some dumbbells have a bubbled-out middle; it's actually thicker in the middle of the handle. This puts more pressure per square inch on part of your hand. This was always a problem for me when using 90s or 100s. A dumbbell with a really thin handle created the same issue, too much pressure on one part of the palm. Most gyms purchase from reputable dumbbell companies who manufacture dumbbells with straight grips that measure just the right thickness.

#2 FOREARM SPLINTS (No, not shin splints, *forearm* splints)

Some weightlifters that go wild on barbell bicep curls may run into this issue. Curling 135 pounds for reps with a 7-foot Olympic straight-bar (used for bench pressing) can be really stressful on not only the biceps, but also the forearm muscles and bone structure. You may find yourself with healed biceps, but sensitive forearms along the bone. They feel just like shin splints if you've run way too much in gym class or track. I remember being so annoyed I couldn't do biceps. Would you believe that this can be solved by just SWITCHING to a CURL BAR? Yes. The change in wrist position takes the pressure off the same spot on the forearm. By the next week, you can do biceps with the straight barbell again.

#3 THE SHOULDER BLADE AND NECK MUSCLE PULL

Sometimes doing an exercise for one muscle has the potential to pull a muscle used to stabilize the exercise movement. Eventually (it took a few times) I realized that during barbell bicep curls, whenever I held the straight bar with my arms shoulder width apart (not wide grip by any means), I would feel a major muscle pull in my neck but mostly along my right shoulder blade. What a joke! Finally I realized my body handled the stress of the weight much better if I grabbed the bar with a slightly narrower grip (where the back of my hands rested against my front-outer thigh muscle at the bottom of the lift). It looks a little strange, but I couldn't argue with my body; it was certainly better than pulling a muscle in my shoulder blade and having to take a week off for it to heal! No thanks. This proves that slight modifications in grips or the way one stands can actually matter. Always pay attention to your grips, stances, and body positions.

SCARY THINGS AND SOME NOT-SO-SCARY THINGS

Everything in life seems to have risks and warnings. Yes, in extreme conditions and rare cases really bad things do happen; however, the odds are against any of this craziness. If you BREATHE while you work out and build slowly, most likely you won't "Die on the Bench" like an older warrior in battle (although I can think of worse ways to go).

#1 HEART ATTACK OR STERNUM PAIN?

Sometimes beginners think they're having a HEART ATTACK. Often, after some major bench pressing, you may feel some pain in the middle of your chest; USUALLY this pain is associated with the heavy bench pressing you did a day or so before. Relax, you're not dying. Even so, definitely pay attention to any pain in your chest and note its location.

#2 SCARY STUFF (PROBABLY EXTREMELY RARE)

All the studies going on in medicine can drive a person crazy. Remember to use common sense and pay attention to your body's signals and you'll probably be fine. Walking around can be a risk. It's best to just be aware of things, but to calm down and realize most people live a long, long time. Here is a list of some crazy topics and issues:

HEART AORTA STRAIN DUE TO LIFTING HEAVY WEIGHTS

(Pay attention if you're always getting lightheaded or nauseated after lifting)

THE POSSIBILITY OF EVENTUALLY DESTROYING MUSCLE PERMANENTLY CALLED "BURNING."

(This seems wildly insane, but who knows . . . .)

DO THIS, DO THAT, DON'T DO THAT

"Drink 64 oz. of water a day! It's good for you! Drinking 64 oz. of water a day is too much. It's bad for you!" Sometimes you might find yourself thinking, "Does *anyone* know what they're talking about?" (Again, you can find medical articles going against each other all the time. One article states that you should lift heavy as an old man, but what about heart strain? Wouldn't this be more dangerous as your whole body ages?) Learn to listen to yourself. Live to lift another day.

RANDOM STUFF AND THE INTERNET

These two things go hand-in-hand. Instead of lifting weights, you can spend countless hours looking up tricks and strategies on the Internet. Nine times out of ten you'll be better off just going to exercise. This is the whole reason for this book. Read it a few times and never look back.

RARELY do breakthroughs in fitness come about. If they do, you'll KNOW ABOUT IT.

It won't cost you three EASY PAYMENTS, monthly payments, be on twenty DVDs, come in some TOTAL equipment solution, be CRAZY FAST, or exist in a BOTTLE, or in two SCOOPS.

Then again, maybe I'm wrong. It just seems to me that growth, good things, and wisdom require a long journey and hard work.

TIME, AGE, AND MUSCLE MEMORY

Try not to think in minutes, days, weeks, or months. Think years. If you're starting a program like this when you're young, you'll have a SIGNIFICANT advantage. It will be easier to stay in shape later in life (or get back into shape). Not only do young people form good habits, but your muscles will "Remember" the intense training they received. This is called "Muscle Memory." It's easier to REGAIN muscle rather than build it for the FIRST TIME.

RISK VS. REWARD

Always determine whether or not the REWARD outweighs the RISK. If you do this, you'll come out ahead of the game every single time. If an exercise such as military press, wherein you press large amounts of weight over your head, doesn't seem worth the stress on your shoulder, don't do it. Why risk trashing your rotator cuff muscles in order to overwork the front shoulder? Why do one-rep-max-outs? You may trash your joints to try to prove your strength. It happens. If you're not becoming a pro arm-wrestler, why do it? It's very hard on the rotator cuff muscles.

GET "HUGE" GET "HIGH"

Lots of kids are missing "feeling good" in their lives. This leads to drugs and other ways to feel good about yourself. Exercising your body causes mental happiness as a side effect, so get HIGH on weightlifting with HUGE as a bonus.

THE RIDDLE OF IRON

We've talked a lot about outer muscle strength and inner core power, but it is important to take a moment to reflect on the mental side of your body. As a once youthful "meathead," I followed a path that led me to believe that injuries were impossible and that every weight was attainable no matter what my genetics. Yes, this willpower can help you through those seemingly impossible reps; however, there must be balance. Eventually, iron will send you its own message; you better listen to it. A great many people from the ancient gyms of past thought they could control iron, pumping as much as they wanted. This is one of the great conundrums of exercise: *The Riddle of Iron*. The secret of iron has always carried with it a mystery. You must learn its riddle. You must learn its discipline. The riddle of iron will always be an enigma that individuals must answer for themselves. I can't tell you what your future picture might look like as a teenager or when you're one hundred years old. The mind and body are amazing things; train them both as long as you can. Learn the riddle of iron and solve it for yourself.

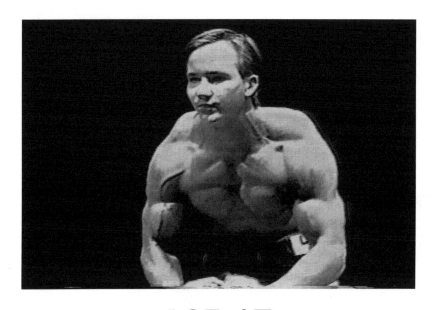

AGE 17

"Live to Lift Another Day!"

APPENDICES

12.

"Fill in the Blanks to Solve the Riddle."

APPENDIX A

(Blank Workout Sheets)

⫶HUGE WORKOUT VERSION "A" ⫶HUGE

DAY 1 (MONDAY) CHEST & BACK

Body Warm-up (slow)   •   5–10 minutes   •   (treadmill, bike, etc.)

(Sets do NOT include a low-weight warm-up set)

Barbell Bench Press	5 sets	8–12 reps	_____ lbs.
Barbell Incline Bench Press	5 sets	8–12 reps	_____ lbs.
Pull-ups (50 reps)	5 sets	8–15 reps	body weight only
Barbell Bent-Over-Row	5 sets	8–12 reps	_____ lbs.

Core Work (Abdominal exercises, planks, etc.)
Rotator Cuff exercises (2–3 sets) (Perhaps with a focus on external cuff muscles.)
Light Stretching
Intensity and reps vary from day-to-day based on soreness, etc. Use common sense and listen to your body.

DAY 2 (TUESDAY) LEGS

Body Warm-up (slow)   •   5–10 minutes   •   (treadmill, bike, etc.)

(Sets do NOT include a low-weight warm-up set)

Squats	5 sets	8–12 reps	_____ lbs.
Leg Press	5 sets	8–12 reps	_____ lbs.
Leg Curls	5 sets	8–12 reps	_____ lbs.
Standing Calf Raises	5 sets	20 reps	_____ lbs.

Core Work (Abdominal exercises, planks, etc.)
Light Stretching
Intensity and reps vary from day-to-day based on soreness, etc. Use common sense and listen to your body.

DAY 3 (WEDNESDAY) ARMS & SHOULDERS

Body Warm-up (slow)   •   5–10 minutes   •   (treadmill, bike, etc.)

(Sets do NOT include a low-weight warm-up set)

Barbell Bicep Curls (standing)	4 sets	8–12 reps	_____ lbs.
Seated Bicep Curls (dumbbells)	4 sets	8–12 reps	_____ lbs.
Overhead Triceps Extension (curl bar)	4 sets	8–12 reps	_____ lbs.
Triceps Pushdown (machine)	4 sets	8–12 reps	_____ lbs.
Side Lateral Shoulder Raises (dumbbells)	5 sets	8–12 reps	_____ lbs.

Core Work (Abdominal exercises, planks, etc.)
Rotator Cuff exercises (2–3 sets) (Perhaps with a focus on external cuff muscles.)
Light Stretching
Intensity and reps vary from day-to-day based on soreness, etc. Use common sense and listen to your body.

WORKOUT VERSION "B"

DAY 4 (THURSDAY) CHEST & BACK

Body Warm-up (slow)   •   5–10 minutes   •   (treadmill, bike, etc.)

(Sets do NOT include a low-weight warm-up set)

Dumbbell Bench Press (dumbbells)	5 sets	8–12 reps	_____ lbs.
Dumbbell Incline Bench Press (dumbbells)	5 sets	8–12 reps	_____ lbs.
Pull-ups (50 reps)	5 sets	8–15 reps	body weight only
Dumbbell Bent-Over-Row (dumbbells)	5 sets	8–12 reps	_____ lbs.

Core Work (Abdominal exercises, planks, etc.)
Rotator Cuff exercises (2–3 sets) (Perhaps with a focus on external cuff muscles.)
Light Stretching
Intensity and reps vary from day-to-day based on soreness, etc. Use common sense and listen to your body.

DAY 5 (FRIDAY) LEGS

Body Warm-up (slow)   •   5–10 minutes   •   (treadmill, bike, etc.)

(Sets do NOT include a low-weight warm-up set)

Squats	5 sets	8–12 reps	_____ lbs.
Leg Press	5 sets	8–12 reps	_____ lbs.
Leg Curls	5 sets	8–12 reps	_____ lbs.
Seated Calf Raises	5 sets	20 reps	_____ lbs.

Core Work (Abdominal exercises, planks, etc.)
Light Stretching
Intensity and reps vary from day-to-day based on soreness, etc. Use common sense and listen to your body.

DAY 6 (SATURDAY) ARMS & SHOULDERS

Body Warm-up (slow) • 5–10 minutes • (treadmill, bike, etc.)

(Sets do NOT include a low-weight warm-up set)

Barbell Bicep Curls (standing)	4 sets	8–12 reps	_____ lbs.
Seated Bicep Curls (dumbbells)	4 sets	8–12 reps	_____ lbs.
One-Arm Triceps Extension (dumbbell)	4 sets	8–12 reps	_____ lbs.
Triceps Pushdown (machine)	4 sets	8–12 reps	_____ lbs.
Side Lateral Shoulder Raises (dumbbells)	5 sets	8–12 reps	_____ lbs.

*Core Work (Abdominal exercises, planks, etc.)
*Rotator Cuff exercises (2–3 sets) (Perhaps with a focus on external cuff muscles.)
*Light Stretching
*Intensity and reps vary from day-to-day based on soreness, etc. Use common sense and listen to your body.

Day 7 (Sunday) OFF

WORKOUT VERSION "C" (WITH PYRAMIDING)

DAY 8 (MONDAY) CHEST & BACK

Body Warm-up (slow) • **5–10 minutes** • **(treadmill, bike, etc.)**

(Low-weight warm-up INCLUDED in 1st set)

Barbell Bench Press	1st set	15 reps	_____ lbs.	
	2nd set	8–10 reps	_____ lbs.	
	3rd set	4–6 reps	_____ lbs.	(The 4th set
	4th set	4–6 reps	_____ lbs.	depends on
	4th set	4–6 reps	_____ lbs.	your level
	4th set	8–10 reps	_____ lbs.	of strength
	5th set	8–10 reps	_____ lbs.	that day.)
	6th set	8–15 reps	_____ lbs.	
Barbell Incline Bench Press	1st set	15 reps	_____ lbs.	
	2nd set	8–10 reps	_____ lbs.	
	3rd set	4–6 reps	_____ lbs.	
	4th set	4–6 reps	_____ lbs.	
	5th set	8–10 reps	_____ lbs.	
	6th set	8–15 reps	_____ lbs.	
Lat Pulldown Machine	1st set	15 reps	_____ lbs.	
	2nd set	8–10 reps	_____ lbs.	
	3rd set	4–6 reps	_____ lbs.	
	4th set	4–6 reps	_____ lbs.	
	5th set	8–10 reps	_____ lbs.	
	6th set	8–15 reps	_____ lbs.	
Barbell Bent-Over-Row	1st set	15 reps	_____ lbs.	
	2nd set	8–10 reps	_____ lbs.	
	3rd set	4–6 reps	_____ lbs.	
	4th set	4–6 reps	_____ lbs.	

	5th set	8–10 reps	_____ lbs.
	6th set	8–15 reps	_____ lbs.

*Core Work (Abdominal exercises, planks, etc.)
*Rotator Cuff exercises (2–3 sets) (Perhaps with a focus on external cuff muscles.)
*Light Stretching
*Intensity and reps vary from day-to-day based on soreness, etc. Use common sense and listen to your body.

WORKOUT VERSION "C"
(WITH PYRAMIDING)

DAY 9 (TUESDAY) LEGS

Body Warm-up (slow) • 5–10 minutes • (treadmill, bike, etc.)

(Low-weight warm-up INCLUDED in 1st set)

Squats	1st set	15 reps	_____ lbs.
	2nd set	8–10 reps	_____ lbs.
	3rd set	4–6 reps	_____ lbs.
	4th set	4–6 reps	_____ lbs.
	5th set	8–10 reps	_____ lbs.
Leg Press	5 sets	8–12 reps	_____ lbs.
Leg Curls	5 sets	8–12 reps	_____ lbs.
Standing Calf Raises	5 sets	20 reps	_____ lbs.

*Core Work (Abdominal exercises, planks, etc.)
*Light Stretching
*Intensity and reps vary from day-to-day based on soreness, etc. Use common sense and listen to your body.

WUGE WORKOUT VERSION "C" WUGE
(WITH PYRAMIDING)

DAY 10 (WEDNESDAY) ARMS & SHOULDERS

Body Warm-up (slow) • 5–10 minutes • (treadmill, bike, etc.)

(Low-weight warm-up INCLUDED in 1st set)

Barbell Bicep Curls (standing)	1st set	15 reps	_____ lbs.
	2nd set	8–10 reps	_____ lbs.
	3rd set	4–6 reps	_____ lbs.
	4th set	8–10 reps	_____ lbs.
Seated Bicep Curls (dumbbells)	4 sets	8–12 reps	_____ lbs.
Overhead Triceps Extension (curl bar)	1st set	15 reps	_____ lbs.
	2nd set	8–10 reps	_____ lbs.
	3rd set	4–6 reps	_____ lbs.
	4th set	8–10 reps	_____ lbs.
Triceps Pushdown (machine)	4 sets	8–12 reps	_____ lbs.
Side Lateral Shoulder Raises (dumbbells)	5 sets	8–12 reps	_____ lbs.

Core Work (Abdominal exercises, planks, etc.)
Rotator Cuff exercises (2–3 sets) (Perhaps with a focus on external cuff muscles.)
Light Stretching
Intensity and reps vary from day-to-day based on soreness, etc. Use common sense and listen to your body.

Day 11 (Thursday) Chest/Back (RESTART with Workout A)

Day 12 (Friday) Legs (RESTART with Workout A)

Day 13 (Saturday) Arms/Shoulders (RESTART with Workout A)

Day 14 (Sunday) OFF

HUGE **NAME** _____ **DATE** _____ **HUGE**

DAY _____ **BODY PART** _____

BODY WARM-UP (TIME) _____**TYPE** _____

EXERCISE | SETS | REPS | WEIGHT

_____   _____   _____   _____

_____   _____   _____   _____

_____   _____   _____   _____

_____   _____   _____   _____

_____   _____   _____   _____

_____   _____   _____   _____

_____   _____   _____   _____

_____   _____   _____   _____

_____   _____   _____   _____

_____   _____   _____   _____

_____   _____   _____   _____

_____   _____   _____   _____

_____   _____   _____   _____

_____   _____   _____   _____

_____   _____   _____   _____

_____   _____   _____   _____

_____   _____   _____   _____

_____   _____   _____   _____

APPENDIX B

(Blank Dieting Sheets)

MEAL # _____

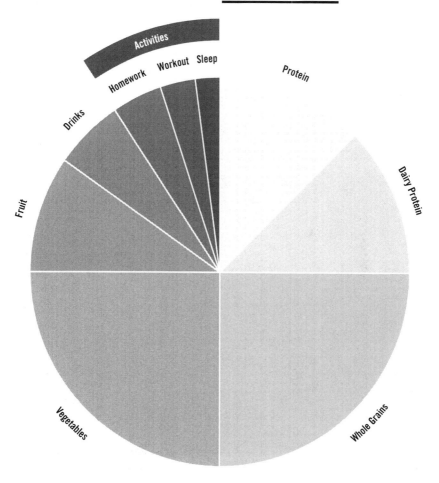

MEAL #1	Calories	Protein	Carbohydrates	Fat
_____	_____	_____	_____	_____
_____	_____	_____	_____	_____
_____	_____	_____	_____	_____
_____	_____	_____	_____	_____
_____	_____	_____	_____	_____

Total =

MEAL #2	Calories	Protein	Carbohydrates	Fat
_____	_____	_____	_____	_____
_____	_____	_____	_____	_____
_____	_____	_____	_____	_____
_____	_____	_____	_____	_____
_____	_____	_____	_____	_____

Total =

MEAL #3	Calories	Protein	Carbohydrates	Fat
_____	_____	_____	_____	_____
_____	_____	_____	_____	_____
_____	_____	_____	_____	_____
_____	_____	_____	_____	_____
_____	_____	_____	_____	_____

Total =

MEAL #4   Calories   Protein   Carbohydrates   Fat

_____   _____   _____   _____   ____

_____   _____   _____   _____   ____

_____   _____   _____   _____   ____

_____   _____   _____   _____   ____

_____   _____   _____   _____   ____

_____   _____   _____   _____   ____

Total =

MEAL #5   Calories   Protein   Carbohydrates   Fat

_____   _____   _____   _____   ____

_____   _____   _____   _____   ____

_____   _____   _____   _____   ____

_____   _____   _____   _____   ____

_____   _____   _____   _____   ____

_____   _____   _____   _____   ____

Total =

MEAL #6   Calories   Protein   Carbohydrates   Fat

_____   _____   _____   _____   ____

_____   _____   _____   _____   ____

_____   _____   _____   _____   ____

_____   _____   _____   _____   ____

_____   _____   _____   _____   ____

Total =

APPENDIX C

(Blank Body Measurement Sheets)

HUGE **NAME** _____   **HUGE**

DATE   _____   DATE   _____

AGE   _____   AGE   _____

HEIGHT   _____   HEIGHT   _____

WEIGHT   _____   WEIGHT   _____

CHEST   _____   CHEST   _____

BICEPS   _____   BICEPS   _____

WAIST   _____   WAIST   _____

LEGS   _____   LEGS   _____

CALVES   _____   CALVES   _____

DATE   _____   DATE   _____

AGE   _____   AGE   _____

HEIGHT   _____   HEIGHT   _____

WEIGHT   _____   WEIGHT   _____

CHEST   _____   CHEST   _____

BICEPS   _____   BICEPS   _____

WAIST   _____   WAIST   _____

LEGS   _____   LEGS   _____

CALVES   _____   CALVES   _____

NAME _____

DATE	_____	DATE	_____
AGE	_____	AGE	_____
HEIGHT	_____	HEIGHT	_____
WEIGHT	_____	WEIGHT	_____
CHEST	_____	CHEST	_____
BICEPS	_____	BICEPS	_____
WAIST	_____	WAIST	_____
LEGS	_____	LEGS	_____
CALVES	_____	CALVES	_____
DATE	_____	DATE	_____
AGE	_____	AGE	_____
HEIGHT	_____	HEIGHT	_____
WEIGHT	_____	WEIGHT	_____
CHEST	_____	CHEST	_____
BICEPS	_____	BICEPS	_____
WAIST	_____	WAIST	_____
LEGS	_____	LEGS	_____
CALVES	_____	CALVES	_____